1 Gram Prot W9-CDE-982

1 Gram Carbo = 4 Cal

1 Gram of Fat = 9 Cal

FAT DESTROYER FOODS:
THE MAGIC METABOLIZER DIET

Sidney Petrie
in association with Robert B. Stone

Foreword by Frank S. Caprio, M.D.

PARKER PUBLISHING COMPANY, INC.
WEST NYACK, N.Y.

Library of Congress Cataloging in Publication Data

Petrie, Sidney.
   Fat destroyer foods.

   1. Reducing diet. I. Stone, Robert B. II. Title.
RM222.2.P45   613.2'5   73-17475
ISBN 0-13-308098-6

Printed in the United States of America

FOREWORD
BY A DOCTOR OF MEDICINE

It is estimated that there are approximately sixteen and a half million Americans who are overweight, and not doing anything about it. This fact alone would justify the need for, and importance of, educating the general public regarding the hazards of obesity—and what they can do to cure themselves of their preoccupation with food that inevitably leads to food addiction and compulsive eating.

Sidney Petrie and Robert B. Stone are to be commended for making available to the lay reader the latest scientific information about weight reduction, and about the "fat destroyer foods" that are used in their "Magic Metabolizer Diet." Their recommended program for weight control has been tested and proved by Petrie's many years of clinical experience in the field, and has helped thousands of overweight men and women of all ages.

As a practicing psychiatrist for over 37 years, I have encountered innumerable cases of persons who, even though they are aware of the health risks of being overweight, continued to eat the wrong foods to excess. Some of them gave up trying to lose their extra poundage and resigned themselves to the inevitable—often succumbing to a premature death.

Petrie, who is psychiatry-oriented and gifted with the ability to establish a positive rapport—a deep empathy—with each client, has included this factor in his overall program for fast weight reduction. His methods help the reader uproot the sub-conscious causes of his fatness, and solve the emotional hang-ups that may be responsible for the compulsion to overeat.

Unfortunately, the majority of people with weight problems are either uninformed or misinformed about the psychic factors that may be contributing to their overweight condition. One of the aims of this book is to dispel common fallacies about food values, diets, caloric intake, and so forth.

For example, the book describes the so-called Yo-Yo Syndrome applicable to those people who lose and gain weight repeatedly. It explains the reason for this, and shows the reader Petrie's practical techniques for overcoming the problem, so that the reader discovers how to lose weight and never gain it back.

In my opinion, the program described by Petrie and Stone in this book, which is built around the "fat destroyer food" diet is medically and psychologically sound, and should prove to be extremely helpful to those who are trying to lose weight if they follow it as directed.

The authors deserve to be congratulated for their dedicated efforts to help their readers develop sensible new eating habits and maintain lifelong weight control.

From cover to cover, I consider this book, in its category, the best I have ever read and I heartily recommend it to anyone who wants to lose weight quickly, easily, automatically and permanently.

As a medical man, I am impressed by the astonishing and dramatic weight loss results achieved by so many of Petrie's patients—even in seemingly hopeless cases referred to him by physicians and other medical specialists.

I am also impressed by Petrie's remarkable discovery of "fat destroyer foods," which I believe to be an entirely new concept in dieting. It permits the dieter to enjoy what I, too, believe is one of the most permissive and pleasant diets ever devised. By scientifically adjusting the body's metabolic processes, these "fat destroyer foods" seem to melt away pound after pound— without debilitating hunger pangs or danger to the body's physical well-being. I can honestly say that, in my medical opinion, this book represents the wave of the future in dieting.

—Frank S. Caprio, M.D.

To my children,
Jacqueline and David
—Sidney Petrie

ACKNOWLEDGMENT

Our heartfelt thanks to Mrs. Gertrude Loris who helped prepare the percentage elements of various foods in this book.

Other Books by the Authors

How to Reduce and Control Your Weight Through Self-Hypnotism
How to Strengthen Your Life with Mental Isometrics
Hypno-Cybernetics: Helping Yourself to a Rich New Life
The Lazy Lady's Easy Diet, a Fast-Action Plan to Lose Weight Quickly for Sustained Slenderness and Youthful Attractiveness
Martinis and Whipped Cream: The New Carbo-cal Way to Lose Weight and Stay Slim
The Miracle Diet for Fast Weight Loss

WHAT YOU HAVE
EVERY RIGHT TO EXPECT
FROM FAT DESTROYER FOODS AND
THE MAGIC METABOLIZER DIET

- Enable you to lose up to five pounds a week without counting calories
- End that "on again, off again" dieting by preventing weight regain
- Keep you feeling that you can lick the world
- Nourish your body better than ever
- Provide three solid meals a day and then some
- Deliver tasteful eating enjoyment all the way
- Cost no more
- Take less food preparation time, not more
- Offer you attractiveness, better health, longer life
- Make you want to shout the news to the rest of the world

Sidney Petrie

WHAT THIS BOOK
CAN DO FOR YOU

The lot of dieters for losing weight has been a sorry one—frazzled nerves, low energy, hunger and martyrdom. The pity is, when your goal is reached, you, the dieter, are so in need of replenishing your weak, starved body you seldom get to enjoy your new-found slenderness before the bulges are back and it's time to go on a diet again.

It is now possible for you to go on a diet that is really not a diet in the old "cut down your food intake" sense. It is a diet that treats your body better than you are probably treating it now. You are fit, alert, and happy. You are never hungry, because your body is never starved. You have all the energy you need, plus vim, vigor, virility, and vitality, and you keep it.

Most diets appear to "work" because they treat the problem on an input-output basis. Eat less calories than you use up each day and your body must consume its own fat. Hardly a month goes by without some "expert" being quoted in newspapers or magazines repeating the "old saw" about cutting down on food intake to lose weight. Yet they keep making the same mistake and pushing their readers, clients, and patients into a common trap:

Less calories on the average diet mean less nutrition, less resistance to disease, less repair to the weary tissues, less mental activity, less physical capability. You get weight loss with this body depletion. But you also get weight gain when the inevitable replenishment of the body occurs.

I have treated thousands of overweight people. At first, I made that same mistake—just cut calories. The lower the calories eaten, the faster people lose weight. It appeared to be a very successful approach.

But then the same people kept coming back year after year. Their weight was up and down. Up and down. It was the same all over the country. Physicians began to call it the "Yo-Yo Syndrome."

The problem was twofold:

1. How can a person be free of hunger and radiantly healthy while dieting?
2. How can a person who gets off a diet stay slim?

I then made a fortuitous discovery.

Certain foods destroy fat! One reason they do so is they provide the body with the vital nutrients it needs to metabolize the fat away. Normal diets deprive the body of these very foods. Another reason is more complicated. Their own metabolism seems to drag body fat with it. You can actually see evidence of your own fat going down the drain.

With these fat destroyer foods, unwanted pounds disappear fast and without hunger pains.

What is just as important, there is no starved body to replenish and no rigid diet to get off. So the 'yo-yo effect is broken and you stay your normal, slim weight.

This is an eat-all-you-want program. Not all you want of celery stalks and lettuce leaves, but all you want of such foods as broiled steak, roast chicken, baked fish, bacon and eggs, gourmet cheeses, and hundreds of other mouth-watering, hunger-satisfying foods.

You need never be on a starvation diet again for weight control. And, without effort or willpower, you can enjoy being the slender, healthy person you know you can and should be. This book shows you how.

Sidney Petrie

Contents

1

WHY STARVATION DIETS ARE NOW OBSOLETE

Some ten years ago, I took time out from my weight control practice to write a book and show how thousands of men and women were losing scores of pounds, effortlessly.

They were not on "diets."

In fact, many were eating more in order to weigh less.

My book, *Martinis and Whipped Cream*,[1] told the truth about carbohydrates.

Apparently, it started a revolution in dieting.

Now we have learned more. It is not only that carbohydrates hang fat on you, but we have found that there are fat destroyer foods that burn it off.

Hundreds of thousands of business men and women, entertainers, models, tycoons—all with one thing in common: unwanted bulges—have slenderized on dinners of roast baron of beef, porterhouse steaks, and shoulder of lamb.

They have lunched regally on broiled mackerel, hamburger steaks, and lobster royal.

They have breakfasted on all the eggs and bacon they could put away.

In addition, they have snacked in between meals, hoisted the elbow at parties, and enjoyed midnight suppers.

---

[1]Parker Publishing Company, Inc., West Nyack, N.Y. © 1966.

While they enjoyed eating, they also enjoyed healthier, slimmer bodies. They found a way to beat the overweight syndrome—permanently.

Now I'm not saying I started this anti-carbohydrate revolution single-handedly. It seems that when an idea's time has come, it receives many helping hands.

A half million of my books are now in print but this is just a drop in the fat bucket compared to the many other good books that have since helped to put the dagger to death-dealing carbohydrates.

I applaud them all.

But there is more good news ahead for dieters . . .

Ways to eat even more.

And lose weight even faster.

The Greatest Dietary Mistake Ever Made by Man

While hundreds of thousands have been adding years to their life expectancy:

- A top university nutritionist calls *Martinis and Whipped Cream* a fraud.
- *Time* magazine in a cover story[2] states disparagingly, "Lovers of martinis, whipped cream or bananas can find diets that emphasize their favorite foods."
- A government nutritionist pot-shots with, "Ever tried a gin and butter diet? Well, please don't."

I have appeared on national television shows, radio talk shows, and have had articles in many popular magazines. Always there crops up built-in opposition to the new idea:

Calories don't count.

It's the kind of calories that count.

But the tide is turning.

When a popular "figure" like formerly rotund Ed McMahon, Johnny Carson's "Tonight Show" sidekick, writes his own book *Slimming Down* and credits my *Martinis and Whipped Cream* program for his success in losing weight. . .

---

[2]December 18, 1972.

When Dr. Stillman makes the bestseller list with *The Doctor's Quick Weight Loss Diet,* then Dr. Fredericks with *Carlton Fredericks' Low Carbohydrate Diet* and Dr. Atkins follows them with *The Diet Revolution . . . .*

Something good for weight loss is happening.

A great error is being corrected.

Whenever this happens, the opponents go through three stages:

    1. "It's crazy."

    2. "It's worth looking into."

    3. "We've known it all along."

I don't think we're at stage three yet.

But we are getting there.

The Greatest Dietary Mistake

The greatest dietary mistake ever made by man is about to be acknowledged.

Whether it will be universally corrected in our time, remains to be seen.

The villain is the carbohydrate.

It has many friends. They all make money on it, or are addicted to it.

The carbohydrate has ascended to a place of undisputed popularity in modern fare. Witness the supermarket breads, rolls, cakes, doughnuts, muffins, pies, and pastry; the dry cereals, crackers and cookies; the pancake mixes, ice creams, waffles, and pizzas.

All are within easy reach of fat fingers, swollen by previous visits.

Primitive man was a protein eater. He seldom consumed any carbohydrates. When he began to till the soil, he shifted to 20 percent to 30 percent carbohydrates in his daily fare.

Today, the situation is reversed, with protein taking a 30 percent back seat to the 70 percent front-running villain, carbohydrate.

Man does not have the ability to metabolize this quantity of carbohydrates.

So a number of things begin to happen: he develops diabetes, or hypoglycemia (low blood sugar), or other metabolic disorders.

Or he merely gets fat.

A beautiful brunette came into my office. I won't mention her name. Even if they generously agree, I don't like to embarrass my clients by perpetuating their overweight pasts. So let's call her L.W. I say beautiful because her face had not puffed up with the rest of her. She was like one of those balloons where the body of the animal inflates but not the head.

Although under 30, she was diabetic and had been taking insulin for four months. "I will not jab that needle in me one more day," she protested.

"You follow your doctor's orders or the interview is over right now," I warned. "But maybe we can get your doctor to change those orders pretty quickly."

Her face lit up. "How?"

I took her eating inventory, part of the initial record-keeping procedure of my office, and I pointed out the carbohydrates that were poisoning her.

"I'll starve to death without them." She seemed on the verge of tears.

"Will you starve to death on Eggs Benedict, Canadian bacon, and Portuguese sausage for breakfast? Cheese soufflé and hamburger steak for lunch? Barbequed spareribs, roast duckling and whipped cream desserts for dinner?"

She left with lists of carbohydrate-free foods,—and obviously suspicious that I was some kind of a "nut," albeit low in carbohydrates.

It took 11 days. Actually, she could have stopped taking the insulin in five or six days according to her blood sugar test. But her doctor played it safe and I agreed with him.

"I have not been hungry for a minute," she reported later.

No hunger—no diet to get on—no diet to get off—no regain of lost weight. That was her experience.

The Yo-Yo Syndrome

Would you care to guess how many times this has happened?

1. A person cuts calories to lose weight.
2. The weight is lost

3. The cut calories are restored.

4. The weight is regained.

Up and down like a yo-yo goes the weight. Some people who are perpetual dieters can lose 50 pounds a year, year in and year out, and yet not vary their weight by more than ten pounds.

A middle-aged client's experience

Here is how a pleasant 54-year old client of mine describes her overweight condition.

"I usually am pretty strong about giving up things that I decide I should give up. I felt that I was having too many cocktails before dinner. I just made the decision to cut down to one with dinner and I was able to stick to it.

"About five years ago when a close friend of mine was struggling to stop smoking, she challenged me to stop if I thought it was so easy. I just did. And when the time was over that I felt was a reasonable test, I just decided there was no sense to going back to smoking so I didn't do it.

"But, I was never able to do that with food. I can cut out certain things. When I became worried about high cholesterol and what foods I shouldn't eat, I was able to get off them. But I don't know what my excess weight is due to, if I eat too much of the wrong foods, or what.

"All my life I've had to diet. I finally go down to a weight that I'm pretty satisfied with and then I just go right on up again. I'm 40 pounds overweight now, and that's too much especially at my age. I am tired of struggling to stay on diets and being hungry all the time."

Every few months some nutritionist comes out with that old axiom: eat less and you'll weigh less.

And that other old axiom: Keep a balanced diet while you lose weight.

What say we put the ax to both axioms right here and now.

I have proved to thousands that they can eat all they want and still lose weight.

I have also proved that a balanced diet—balanced with carbohy-drates according to present day standards—can be a *killer*.

Whenever I read some article about how to lose weight by getting the proper exercise and eating a balanced diet, I wonder whether the "authority" believes what he is really saying.

He is dooming the gullible reader to the yo-yo syndrome.

He is prescribing hunger to shrink fat cells.

He is prescribing an end to hunger to restore fat cells.

The Carbohydrate "Conspiracy"

It seems as if there were some giant conspiracy going on. I'm not saying there is, but it certainly looks that way.

Compare the carbohydrate to hard drugs.

There are the "pushers" and the addicts.

The carbohydrate pushers are the food processers who keep finding new carbohydrate products to push.

You and I become addicts because:

1. Carbohydrates are quick and easy foods.

2. Carbohydrates taste good as food should.

The carbohydrate pushers use sugar to hook us.

They tantalize us, when we are toddlers, with sweet goodies that pacify and reward us.

Then it is easy to go on to sugared cereals, sugared doughnuts, sweet chocolates and candy bars, sweet drinks and sugar on the table to add to anything they've overlooked.

Possibilities of a Protein "Conspiracy"

Suppose there was a protein "conspiracy" instead of a carbohydrate "conspiracy."

Sugar cane growers and wheat farmers might shift to grazing cattle or raising poultry. Sugar and grain refiners would convert to slaughterhouses and meat packaging plants, to cheese, dairy and egg wholesalers. Many truck farmers would shift from potatoes and starchy vegetables to the lower-in-carbohydrates leafy kind.

Soft drink bottlers would come up with a whole new line of high-protein throat refreshers. Snack makers might invent ways of packaging slices of filet mignon, or pressed duck.

And you know what?
We'd all be slimmer.
Feel younger.
Work better.
Love more.
And live longer.

Gone would be the obesity industry that thrives on the sale of diet pills, so-called diet foods, and every gadget imaginable from corsets to heat boxes to vibrators. Gone would be the diet books. (I'll gladly make that sacrifice.) Gone would be 90 percent of the overweight specialists. (No sacrifice for me here as I help people to change *all* unwanted habits.)

I'm sorry, though. It's not going to happen . . . really.

You Can Start Your Own Protein Revolution

If you want to end the carbohydrate conspiracy and start a protein revolution, you will have to do it in your own life, or at most, that of your family.

I promise you will find it easy to do and rewarding in many ways.

You will begin to enjoy eating more than ever before as your taste buds broaden their sweets-limited horizons.

You will feel more vital as your body responds to fat destroying foods—foods that, while they destroy fat, build healthy tissue, organs, bone, muscle, skin, and hair.

How Mrs. B.F. ran her protein revolution

B.F. was 39 years young. She was married, had two grown children and worked as a nurse for a doctor who had referred a number of his obesity patients to my office. She was 35 pounds overweight the day she decided to refer herself. Being a nurse and associated with a physician, she had tried appetite depressants and diuretics (to squeeze the water out of her body) on and off for a period of four years. All she got, besides a ride on the yo-yo, were heart palpitations, often caused by appetite depressants, and pains in her ankles and wrists, often caused by diuretics.

Her diet proved to be average American. In other words, pretty bad. But still we had to make only a few switches:

- Bacon and eggs took the place of breakfast Danish pastries.
- Hamburger steaks took the place of luncheon hamburger sandwiches.
- Salads took the place of bread and potatoes at dinner.
- Melon and cheese cake replaced layer cake and pie.

During the first week—without skipping a mouthful—she lost three pounds. After that, she leveled off at about two pounds a week and in four months, she was at her best weight.

Take a look at those substitutions. She was switched to a diet of 95 percent proteins. She received a few carbohydrates in the salads, cheese dessert, and melon. But there are no carbohydrates in meat, eggs, fish, poultry and cheese.

The Vital Material Your Body Cannot Manufacture

Suppose I told you that your body needs three kinds of foods. Let's call them Food A, B, and C.

Now suppose I told you that your body could turn A into B or B into A. But it could not turn either A or B into C.

Which of the three foods would you consider most vital? If your body can get A from B or B from A, but it can get its supply of C only from C, why, of course, C becomes very important.

Now, suppose I was to tell you that practically the entire structure of the body was made of C—hair, skin, veins, flesh, cartilage, organs, intestines, brain, etc. How important is C now? And if I also told you the body could change C into B or A if it needed to, doesn't C grow even more important?

The way most people eat you'd think C stood for carbohydrate.

It stands for protein. The A, B, C's of food are carbohydrate, fat, and protein.

Protein *is* your body. And your body cannot manufacture it.

Most cells of your body are renewed every year—even bone cells. Your body depends on protein foods for this rebuilding.

You can eat five thousand calories of fats and carbohydrates every day for a year. Yet, you can starve to death doing it.

Is it any wonder that Mrs. Dieter, who goes on a regimen of grapefruit, melba toast, tomato aspic, consommé, one lamb chop, watercress and tea, is hungry?

Her skin cells are crying for replacements.

Her brain cells are working overtime.

Her muscle cells are depleted.

Her nails are softening.

Her hair is getting ready to fall out.

Her kidneys, spleen, liver, heart and lung cells are screaming for regeneration.

How long can she keep it up? Not very long.

Result: paradise lost, poundage regained.

What Are Fat Destroyer Foods?

A moment ago, I pointed out that the body can create fat and carbohydrate even though you feed it only protein.

Carbohydrate is the body's fuel. It needs carbohydrate to keep it warm and mobile.

Fat is the body's way of storing fuel.

When you consume carbohydrate foods, the body either utilizes them immediately for heat and energy, or it stores them for future use by converting them to fat.

When you consume fats and oils, the body either converts them into carbohydrates for heat and energy or stores them for future use.

When you consume proteins, the body utilizes them for rejuvenation or converts them into either carbohydrate for energy or fat for storage.

The old school of nutrition has stood four square on the theory that total energy of food intake—measured by the calories—must equal total energy expended if weight is to remain stable.

They have asserted, ever since the rather limited studies of Drs. Johnson and Newburgh at the University of Michigan in 1930, that the calories you eat minus the calories you expend determines whether you lose or gain.

Any engineer who looks at the body as a heat-work machine can punch holes in this calorie statement. He sees other inputs and other outputs.

He sees the input of some 30,000 breathing inhalations a day and the output of an equivalent number of exhalations. These must be examined for differences in energy.

He sees the input and output of water, the latter through the pores as well as the kidneys.

He sees output of solid wastes as a variable—through the pores, the bladder and bowels.

The calorie-in, calorie-out concept could be true if the whole person was isolated and his environment measured along with his body. But things happen to his exhalation, his urine and his excrement that the calorie-in, calorie-out concept ignores.

FACT: Urine, excrement, and exhalations change when there is a diet shift from carbohydrate-*heavy* to protein-*heavy*.

You can check this FACT for yourself:

Step 1 Buy a package of urine test sticks or tablets at your local drug store. These sticks or tablets turn purple when ketones are present in the urine. Test your urine.

Step 2. Shift to a diet totally free of carbohydrates, heavy in protein.

Step 3. Test your urine that same day and the subsequent day.

Within twenty-four hours of going off carbohydrates and on proteins, your sticks or tablets should begin to turn purple, showing the presence of ketones.

Ketones are the by-product of fat being destroyed. If they are in your urine, chances are they are in your breath, too.

Each ketone contains energy that was being stored as fat hours before.

Does the old "tried and true" calorie-in, calorie-out concept begin to sound like "the earth is flat?"

I'm not making myself out to be a Christopher Columbus because I am in no way the first to discover the error of this calorie concept.

Many others have now confirmed that *when you cut out carbohydrates, your body excretes hundreds and hundreds of calories a day extra.*

These excreted calories are fat—unwanted fat in the process of being destroyed.

FACT: Eat protein and fat, with the absolute minimum of carbohydrate, and you destroy your own unwanted fat.

How Fat Is Destroyed When You
Substitute Proteins for Carbohydrates

It was not until 1960 that scientists discovered that when there were no carbohydrates in the diet, the body was triggered to emit a hormone that literally mobilized the body to burn its own fat.

It happened at Middlesex Hospital in London, where Professor Alan Kekwich and Doctors G.L.S. Pawan and T.M. Chalmers isolated a fat destroying hormone in the urine of patients on carbohydrate-free diets but found no evidence of this hormone when carbohydrate was placed in the diet even in small amounts.

This is the hormone that makes the difference.

This is the reason why the no-carbohydrate and low-carbohydrate diets succeed.

You can thank your lucky pituitary gland for your now being able to restore your weight to normal without starving.

The old guard cry is, "Let the overweight now under-eat. Let the punishment fit the crime."

Instead, the new cry is, "Let the overweight now eat protein instead of the carbohydrate that puts the pounds on them."

In a way, the punishment still fits the crime. If you can call it punishment to. . .

- Substitute dry wine for sweet wine or beer.
- Substitute gravy for breads and stuffing.
- Substitute salad for potato.
- Substitute cream soups and clear soups for flour-thickened soups.
- Substitute roasts for pastas.
- Substitute zabaglione or crème de mocha for pie or cake.

Is the No Carbohydrate Diet Right for You?

I have had remarkable success with my clientele for over 20 years of carbohydrate cutting.

However, I have one requirement and I make this a requirement for you, the reader, too:

Remain under the supervision of your doctor while changing your eating regimen

The reason for this requirement is that everybody is different. No regimen can be right for everybody.

Despite the remarkable results you can achieve on the no carbohydrate diet, you need to play it safe and have your family physician examine you as you progress.

There's a shop in London called "Anything Lefthand, Ltd."

It carries a hundred or more items ranging from left-handed can openers to left-handed golf clubs, playing cards, and even billfolds. With some 300 million sinistrals—the technical name for lefties—in the world, the shop does a booming mail order business.

Though I have seen only rare cases where high protein diets have run into metabolic imbalances, I know there must be millions of people who, because of their special health histories, must seek some other approach.

To satisfy your special needs, I have provided you with the diets I give my special clients. These are in Chapters 9 and 10. One is a remarkable sandwich diet. The other is a versatile rice diet. Both require discipline. There is no such thing as "eat all you want." If your doctor so orders, you might as well skip over to Chapters 9 and 10 right now.

The rest of you hundred million overweight people who are ready to get on an abundant protein fare—and off the starvation diet tread mill once and for all—read on.

There are progressive steps for continuing a protein-conscious program so as to continue and even accelerate weight loss. It is like shifting gears in a car. There are special detours, too, for special people. Harriet was one.

A case history in point

Harriet, a telephone operator, 34 years old, divorced, and an impressive 5 feet 10 inches tall, was one of those many who come to me "as a last resort." With tears in her eyes, she told me how her doctor had given her up in despair. She felt she had come to me with her doctor's blessings because he had told her that he did not care where she went and what she tried so long as she lost weight.

She had been on starvation diets, crash diets, diet pills, and anything else that offered promise of weight loss. She did lose weight each time, (does that strike a familiar note with you?) but invariably after she returned to what she called "normal eating," she gained weight again, and in each instance, more than she had lost.

An analysis of her diet showed that she ate all the wrong foods: spaghetti, lasagna, pizza, in fact all sorts of pie, ice cream, and pastries.

I guess you're wondering how much Harriet weighed. At the time of her marriage she had weighed 320 pounds. This was her lowest weight as an adult. After the birth of her child and her divorce, her weight began to climb. Apparently, her unhappiness and depressed state of mind caused her to over-overeat. She reached a point when food was constantly on her mind. She felt, as she put it, as if she had turned into a "food addict."

My scale, which had a maximum capacity of 400 pounds, did not register her weight. This proved that she weighed more than 400 pounds the day she came in. Her dress size was 60.

Harriet's basic problem

She had a water retention problem. Therefore, with the approval of her doctor, I put her on my Rice Diet (see Chapter 10). When she came for her next visit, she claimed that she had lost at least ten pounds. We tried the scale again, but it still did not budge. Obviously, she was still over 400 pounds.

The next step was my Free Diet (see Chapter 3). She followed it faithfully although it banned all her favorite foods. With the loss of the first ten pounds, she had tasted success and was now determined to go all the way.

Harriet's progress

A short time later the scale registered 398 pounds. A substantial weight loss was registered week after week. She had come to me in January, and in June of the same year, I reported to her physician a total weight loss of 120 pounds without any ill effects on her health. She, herself, was particularly impressed with the fact that she never felt hungry and was not at all tempted to eat between meals.

As her weight loss continued very satisfactorily, I started spacing her visits further apart to prepare her for the time when she would have to monitor her food intake without my supervision. The result was most gratifying. When she was close to her right weight, I changed her diet to my Protein Maintenance Diet (Chapter 12). Harriet, today, is remaining her attractive, statuesque self—sans hunger.

"No" Carbohydrate Versus "Low" Carbohydrate

Ten years ago, most of us dealing with weight loss, who knew about the villainy of carbohydrates, still had a healthy respect for this food and its place in the body's metabolism.

We knew that to cut carbohydrates down to zero accelerated the loss of weight but also upset the acid-alkaline balance of the system. Acidosis was the sword of Damocles that we tended to avoid.

Today, we don't look upon the purple of the acetones showing in urine tests as seriously as we did then. We accept the acid system as a temporary condition indicative of the result we aim for: destruction of fat.

The "old" carbohydrate limit

At that time we set 60 grams of carbohydrate as the maximum allowance for a weight loss program. This is about 250 carbohydrate calories.

To somebody who has been on a no-carbohydrate program, this sounds like a lot. Yet, 250 carbohydrate calories (carbo-cals) can be exceeded in one day with:

1/2 medium grapefruit	72
2 slices of white bread	96
1 8-oz. cup of split pea soup	96
	264 carbo-cals

You are also over your 250 daily carbo-cals with:

1 cup freshly squeezed Florida orange juice	98
1 medium baked potato	80
1 medium ear of corn	120
	298 carbo-cals

Now, 250 carbo-cals are too many for some people. They have to substitute proteins almost all the way.

The delightful aspect of this is that you don't have to limit yourself to substituting only 250 protein calories of meat, fish or poultry for 250 carbohydrate calories of sweets and starches.

You can profit hundreds of calories and still lose weight.

Give up the grapefruit, bread and pea soup and add:

Three fried eggs	6	300
Broiled bluefish (medium)	0	195
American cheese (1 oz.)	1	100
	7 carbo-cals	595

You have added about 300 total calories but you will very likely lose faster. The important factor is you have eliminated 257 carbohydrate calories, cutting down these "fat hooks" to where there are no more left for your fat to hang on. In their place, you have put fat destroyer proteins.

So it is metabolized away, urinated away, breathed away.

A young person's problem

Miss L.J. was a telephone operator. She was 23 when she came to see me and weighed 160 pounds—on the increase. She was very cooperative. She carried her carbo-cal tables with her and conscientiously stayed under 200 carbo-cals. In several months she was down to 125 pounds—no starvation, no sweat.

Then she changed jobs. Her new job required her to bring her lunch to work. In her first month, she gained three pounds. Of course, it was the sandwich she was now bringing for lunch. She figured in one year she would regain all the weight she lost. She called me. I recommended that she freeze chicken salad or shrimp salad the night before so that when she took it to work it would be thawed out by lunch. She stopped gaining and soon lost those three pounds. It all pivoted on 100 calories. And they did not have to be cut out, only changed from carbohydrate to protein.

The Choice of the Carbohydrate Program

It is up to you (and your physician) whether you decide to go on a "no" carbohydrate or "low" carbohydrate program, that is, a high protein program or a still higher protein program.

If the progress is unsatisfactory, you can substitute more proteins for carbohydrates until the fat begins to melt away.

A middle-aged married man's problem solved

Ronald was a happily married, successful business man in his early 40's, father of two boys and a girl. He tipped the scales at 305 pounds, some 130 pounds overweight! His weight had never concerned him very much and probably never would have if his doctor had not strongly emphasized the possibility of a heart attack if he did not lose a sizable amount of weight.

Ronald enjoyed food, particularly pastas, bread, cake, pie, and he liked his glass of wine, especially sweet wine, with a stronger drink now and then. I wondered how I could get his weight down and still have him retain his jovial attitude and light-hearted demeanor.

I started by giving him my Highest Protein (Crash) Diet (see Chapter 5) in the hope that the time limitation to which it is subject would present less strain for him. I could then shift him to a more permissive diet. To my surprise, he accepted this crash diet quite readily. He lost 12 pounds during the first week. He felt quite proud of himself, explaining that it really had not been any hardship because he had considered it a game he was playing with himself.

When I put him on my Free Diet (Chapter 3), he followed with the same good-humored attitude. There followed a steady weight loss, week after week, and in five months he had lost 58 pounds. He obviously became "conditioned" to the new way of eating and continued to show satisfactory progress towards his weight goal of 175 pounds without any adverse effect on his disposition, and certainly not on his general health In about 15 months he reached his goal and was an even happier man than he had been before. The last I heard he was on my Protein Maintenance Diet (see Chapter 12) and keeping his doctor happy, too.

Home Sweet Home (for Fat Building)

It's a typical American home, presented to you as follows: There is a glass jar of hard candies on the coffee table and a box of chocolate covered peppermints on the TV console.

In the kitchen, there are cookies in the cookie jar and three different frozen cakes or pies in the freezer. The freezer is also stocked with a quart of butterscotch ice cream, frozen rolls and cans of fruit juice, many with sugar added.

In the refrigerator, are cans of soda and beer with more handy packs stacked behind the door, waiting their turn.

Home sweet home,—starchy but stocked. No having to run down to the corner store because you're out of potato chips; there's another big bag in the cabinet.

You've decided that you are as overstuffed as the furniture and you want to lose weight. If you live alone, it's a relatively easy matter. You clean house—gift your neighbors with the cans, jars, and packages of goodies.

If you do not live alone, you have a "relative" problem. You are not going to be able to easily alter your environment as a means of insulating yourself from the sweet and starchy scoundrels, unless you can convince the family it is as right for them as it is for you.

Let's assume that you are the about-to-be enlightened one and that the rest of the household are not yet convinced of what sweets and starches are doing to them.

I am going to give you right here and now a way you can build up a strong resistance to the siren call of the sugary rascals and starchy scoundrels. If you follow these instructions, you will be able to walk by those TV peppermints and never see them, open the refrigerator door and look right through the soda, watch John eating butterscotch ice cream and, if anything, be revolted by it.

How to Turn Your Mind Away
From Carbohydrate Foods (It's Easy)

Here is what I want you to do.

- Sit comfortably in a chair.
- Close your eyes.
- Visualize a package of potato chips or pretzels or a favorite carbohydrate snack that is likely to remain around the house.
- See yourself opening up the package, placing some in your mouth, chewing, swallowing.
- See the material descend your throat, enter your stomach and turn to fat.
- See yourself bulging with that ugly fat.
- See the fat interfere with proper functioning of your vital organs.
- See the fat bringing you unwanted circumstances.
- Now see yourself refusing to open that package again.
- See yourself, instead, helping yourself to some tuna fish or a chicken leg.

Now don't expect to get any good out of reading the above.

You have to put the book down and you must use the visualizing power of your mind to see the "action" step by step as described.

Put the book down now and do it.

The good you can accomplish for yourself

What you have just done is to reinforce your resolve to "make a change." Even if your family shoves the formerly tempting sweet in front of you, it will no longer tempt you.

This mental exercise works best—

1. The more relaxed you are.
2. The more vivid your mental picture.
3. The more frequently you repeat the exercise.

What you are really doing is starting a mental reprogramming. It is one of the healthiest actions you can take right now.

Later, as you begin to enjoy succulent meats and roasts and poultry and eggs and cheeses, you will be forming new habits. There will be no conscious effort to it.

The important thing is to see yourself as a "protein-arian." See yourself eating abundantly of fat destroying steaks, chops, roasts, shellfish, fish steaks, poultry, eggs and cheeses.

Understand the fat producing role of carbohydrates in your life.

Consider carbohydrates as poison to your system.

See carbohydrates as the hooks that hang pounds on you.

Know that just a mouthful of sweet or starch can hang a pound of flesh on your abdomen, legs, hips, or buttocks.

"Pass the spareribs again, please . . . "

Why Some Protein Foods Destroy Fat
Faster Than Others

A typical case of a middle-aged sedentary male

Henry, a high-school principal was, at 46, tipping the scales at 300 pounds. At 20 he had been a vigorous young man, rather large boned, energetic and his 6'1" frame was an asset to his college football team.

He had always tended to be heavy but his athletic activities kept his muscles lean and taut and although he had a ferocious appetite, his college weight remained reasonably stable at 180-190 pounds. During a particularly strenuous play, he suffered a severe injury to his back which terminated his football career. Almost immediately, he began to add weight. By the time he was 30, he had gained 60 pounds and although he weighed 300 pounds at the time of my initial interview, he had previously reached as high as 330 pounds.

During the period of his conventional dieting, he was able to lose (and regain) weight quite rapidly. But he found it quite difficult to judge his caloric intake on these calorie-restricting diets. He also failed on diets that had a type of food that he liked but which was strictly limited or prohibited.

What Henry accomplished

In the first month of my High Protein Diet (see Chapter 4), he lost 30 pounds and continued to lose weight steadily until he had returned to 190 pounds.

At no time did he run into the difficulties that he had experienced in his former diets. Nor did he complain at any time that he was hungry or that he felt deprived and, as an additional bonus, the back pains that had plagued him since his accident completely disappeared.

Once we realize that we can eat all we want and still lose weight—providing we skirt around carbohydrates—then we are able to pick and choose the best proteins.

The "Best" Proteins

By the best proteins I mean the kind that are lower in fat and higher in minerals, vitamins, and other nutrients.

Some nutritionists and obesiologists are "hung up" on fat. They have been taught that fat causes fat. They often feel it is more important to cut out fat than to cut out carbohydrates.

Also, they differ on the importance of minerals and vitamins. Some prescribe massive doses of vitamins and recommend certain supplements. Others feel that the minimum daily requirements are available—even in reduced food intake.

I am not too concerned with fatty foods. If you have the choice of lean meats instead of meats with a high fat content, of course, I vote lean. But one hundred extra calories of fat are not going to interfere with your weight loss one fraction of the amount that one hundred calories of carbohydrates will.

Vitamins and minerals as useful tools in paring fat

As to vitamins and minerals, I see them as useful tools to the body in destroying fats. The fat destroying hormone, triggered when proteins arrive without carbohydrates, needs minerals and other nutrients to complete the fat destroying process.

We are accustomed to obtaining many of these vitamins and minerals from starchy fruits and vegetables which we are no longer going to eat. So we need to be aware of the best proteins, the proteins richest in nutrients, to keep us at a high level of nutrition, free of the kinds of hunger we often experience on the usual diet.

These best proteins are the best fat destroying foods.

But all proteins are your friends.

All carbohydrates are your enemies.

Warning!

It won't be easy to turn your back on carbohydrates.

They pull you with sweet memories.

They reach out to you from transparent packages.

"Bet you can't eat just one."

They call to you through the voices of radio and television commercials.

They bombard your senses all day long.

What you must now do is drown out this bombardment. Be ready to fight the sweet with the savory, the rich in starch with the rich in flavor.

Get ready to drown out the insidious call of carbo-cals with the sizzling sounds of pleasurable proteins.

And watch your weight melt away.

2

EAT LAVISHLY OF FAT BURNING FOODS
AND STILL LOSE WEIGHT

Children in poor families tend to be fatter than their richer cousins. A study of some three thousand youngsters in Philadelphia, Wilmington, and New York showed that while 29 percent of girls from lower socio-economic levels were obese at age six, only 3 percent of upper level girls had an overweight problem at this age. In the case of the six-year old boys it was 40 percent for the lower brackets, 25 percent for the higher income brackets.

The study did not go into causes, but it is a good bet that if it did, it would find carbohydrates raising their ugly head.

Cereal, bread, potatoes, spaghetti, rice—these are cheap foods, easy on tight budgets but tough on tight clothes.

Wherever carbohydrates abound, obesity is a way of life. The director of East Germany's Central Institute for Nourishment recently reported that 20 percent of the men and 40 percent of the women there were at least 20 percent overweight. Hawaiians who dote on poi, a paste of the starchy taro root, pride themselves on their rotundity.

"Let them eat cake," Marie Antoinette's notorious advice to her starving subjects, would have been more valid as, "Let them eat steak."

The less you eat, the more you lose, will be forever true,—with one exception.

38

Switch from carbo-cals to prote-cals and you will lose more even if you eat more.

The Real Cost of Protein Eating

Will a protein diet cost more?

On the face of it, yes. In the long run, no.

A couple who switched from the average flake and cake daily menu to one featuring steak—ground, potted, or broiled—found that they added $12 to their weekly food budget. The weight they lost cost them an average of $2 per pound each. Later, it even cost them $8 to $10 per week to remain on a high protein maintenance program.

But their doctor's bills went down. They looked better at their optimum weight. They felt younger, more energetic, more enthusiastic.

Can you put a price on that?

You don't have to eat steak seven days a week, chopped, flank or otherwise. Chicken, beef liver, and canned tuna are excellent fat destroying foods and are reasonably enough priced to fit modest budgets.

I admit there is a direct cost for the privilege of eating the way you like to while you lose weight. Proteins cost more than carbohydrates. But the whole problem of overweight can be so costly the way most people are handling it that this differential is really quite a minor matter.

Most doctors make the truth about losing weight hard to swallow. They tend to get you involved in endocrinology and amphetamines and metabolism.

Losing weight is not as easy as pie but it is as easy as shish kebab or beef stroganoff.

Forget the whole idea of going on a diet.

Just go on an anti-carbohydrate, pro-protein campaign.

Then watch what happens to your weight.

Psychologically Speaking, Diets Are Contra-Indicated

Have you ever come across drug ads in medical journals?

"Contra-indicated," they might read, "Known hypersensitivity to the drug; children under two years of age; tendency to urinary retention; acute narrow angle glaucoma; should not be given within two weeks of treatment with a monoamine oxidase inhibitor."

For many drugs the negative contra-indications, side effects, precautions and warnings are five times as lengthy as the positive advantages!

Suppose conventional melba toast and carrot stick starvation diets were required to spell out their contra-indications. They might read like this:

- Should not be administered without continuous professional counsel and reassurance.
- Watch for frequent side effects such as drowsiness and fatigue.
- Acute tension may result from removal of sedative effects of frequent eating.
- Severe depression and frequently immobilizing psychoneurotic anxiety are possible side effects.
- Guilt and self-incrimination, sometimes accompanied by suicidal tendencies, can result from inability to adhere to diet requirements.

The list could go on and on.

It could refer to the danger to vital organs when diets are stopped and started again and the body is subjected to cycles of weight loss and weight regain.

It could point to the surfacing of acute psychological hang-ups that have required food to keep them in a state of quiescence.

It could list physical symptoms that are likely to be aggravated by low calorie regimens.

And indeed these factors could very well apply to a degree on the sandwich diet and rice diet spelled out in Chapters 9 and 10. However, I have selected these diets for special clients who cannot tolerate a high protein diet because the bread and rice diets are, in my opinion, the least difficult.

The Secret of Success of
Successful Weight Losing Organizations

One of the reasons that organizations, such as TOPS (Take Off

Pounds Sensibly) and Weight Watchers, are so successful is that the group provides the individual with the psychological reinforcement that a rigid diet demands.

Actually, the diet that Weight Watchers promotes is one that anybody could get by walking into a New York City Health Department obesity clinic. But what gives the organization its prime value to the dieter is the sympathetic counseling from other members when the going gets rough and the applause and admiration when the pounds come off.

A diet can be a traumatic or dreadful experience.

If you belong to a group, you can share the agony.

The pity of it all is that, for those who go on a strict diet where the main ingredient is deprivation, there is a built-in failure factor:

Stop dieting—start regaining your ideal weight (and shape).

Don't Diet—Just Direct

There is no diet in this book.

Yes, there are menus and recipes and lists of carbo-cals and prote-cals.

The purpose of these is not to enable you to diet, that is to *slow* your eating. Rather it is to *direct* your eating.

The big difference

There's a big difference in directing your diet as given in this book.

If you can continue to eat all you want, *you don't have to worry* about all those psychological contra-indications, warnings, side effects and precautions.

You don't have to worry about *hunger.* You don't have to worry whether or not you will be morally strong enough to exert the *will power* needed to succeed.

You won't be hungry. You won't need will power.

You won't need a group of people to hold your hand or slap you on the back for encouragement. Instead, friends will come to you to find out how you are able to eat so well and still lose so much.

A cartoon shows a patient on a scale in a doctor's office. The doctor is saying, "I'm taking you off sugar 'n spice and everything nice."

That's a non-directed diet, albeit exaggerated in the interests of humor.

"I'm taking you off sugar, starch and sweet, but you can stay on spices and meals of protein complete."

That's a directed diet.

Diet, though, is a misnomer. If you can eat all you want of the right foods, that's a directed eating regimen or program.

What a difference directed eating makes, instead of dieting, to your nerves, well-being, disposition, and personality!

Instead of fading, you bloom.

Exceptions

Now there are some rare exceptions.

Newspaper wire services recently ran an item about a 38-year old man who was eating himself to death, purposely. At the age of 20 he had been a drug addict, which apparently triggered a self-destruction drive. He became obsessed with food. His weight went up by the hundreds of pounds. In 1971, it reached a peak of 1,187 pounds. He was a sideshow attraction in carnivals and fairs where he made speeches against the use of drugs. Then he accepted psychiatric treatment and has since lost over 250 pounds. Even so, at 900 pounds, he occasionally gets acutely ill and doctors need a crane and fork lift truck to move him. If he is reading this book, he should forget it and stick with his psychiatrist.

Bozo's case of exceptional eating

The Guinness Book of Records notes that a man named Bozo has been undefeated in eating contests since 1931. Among his gustatory feats it records, are 27 pullets, each weighing two pounds, consumed at one sitting. And, would you believe, 324 ravioli at another. Now 63, Bozo lives in California. A framed motto in his living room says, "Nothing exceeds like excess."

If Bozo, or any other "excessive" people are reading this book, put it down and go back to the table.

There are some factors, more critical than being overweight, that eclipse that problem.

We are talking in this book, not to these special areas, but to Mr., Mrs. and Miss Average Person who wants to be slender and stay that way—without dieting.

You Can Keep Your Psychological Hang-Ups on This Program

It's an old story—people overeat because of *emotional reasons*. These reasons can be boiled down to one word—fear.

Here are some common fears that drive men and women to food and drink:

Fear of illness.
Fear of losing a job.
Fear of sex.
Fear of no sex.
Fear of people in authority.
Fear of being criticized.
Fear of feeling disapproval from others.
Fear of being ignored or left out.
Fear of being bullied.
Fear of speaking to groups.
Fear of being raped.
Fear of getting pregnant.
Fear of dark places.
Fear of insomnia.
Fear of God.
Fear of responsibility.
Fear of failing.

What happens to somebody who is used to quieting his fear of losing a job by having a big meal when that big meal is refused him? He is bothered by more than hunger. He succumbs quickly, not because of weak will power, but because he is frantic for food. It is his palliative, his tranquilizer, his only relief. With the no-carbohydrate diet, there are no frantic moments for the fear-ridden. Eat all you want when you need it most. The starvation low-calorie diets seem worse than Inquisition tortures. But you can keep your fears and anxieties on this program. Lose weight first. Tackle hang-ups later.

How to Recognize Eat-All-You-Want Proteins When You See Them

I am now going to direct your attention to foods that you can eat all you want of and still lose weight.

In the process, I hope I will be directing your appetite and your craving, too. I don't mind damning carbohydrates, but rather than keep talking about what you should not eat and giving you more of the old "don't" business that you've heard only too often, I'd rather sing the praise of delicious protein foods that destroy fat as you enjoy all you want of them.

Picture these foods as I describe them. They are familiar to you. Recall moments of pleasure when you particularly remember the way so-and-so prepared this dish, or how it was served at such-and-such restaurant. Visualize how you would enjoy some right now. These are foods that have few or no carbohydrates. Some may have a trace, but in no way is this enough to interfere with your weight loss.

Breakfasts

Let's start with *breakfast*.

Eggs are Americans' traditional breakfast food. Are you limited to one medium boiled egg? Absolutely not. Have two large ones, even three, and if you feel you must have four don't let your conscience bother you. You will still lose weight that day.

What's more you can boil them hard, medium or soft. You can fry them, scramble them or poach them. You can make an omelette if you feel like cooking—mushroom or Spanish. Or even Eggs Benedict, but without the English muffins. And if you want to get real fancy, how about shirred eggs (baked) or baked eggs Gruyere (with cheese)?

Some surprising news

If you have toast with your eggs, you have blown it. Goodbye weight loss today, and maybe tomorrow, too.

If you are accustomed to cooking scrambled eggs with a dash of milk, use a teaspoonful of heavy cream instead. You heard right. There are less carbo-cals in cream than milk.

Bacon with the eggs? Sure thing! Thin sliced, thick sliced, and as many slices as you like. Canadian bacon or ham are fine, too. So are link sausages, Portuguese sausage, and other varieties so long as they don't have grain fillers in them. Scrapple is an example of a taboo breakfast "meat." Actually, it is only part meat—scraps of pork boiled with a mixture of meal or flour.

Tripe is popular in some parts of the country as a breakfast food. It is all protein. The English like kippered herring for breakfast or shad roe—all fish are protein. Veal kidneys are a favorite with many—a real fat destroyer food. Any organ meat is rich in protein and minerals and devoid of nasty carbohydrate. Hash with potatoes is a "no-no."

Lunches

Now for *lunch* . . .

Since ease of preparation—even lack of preparation—is the key to the noonday meal, let's spotlight the quickies.

All of the breakfast foods just mentioned are, of course, in the eat all you want category for lunch, too. Lunch also dovetails with dinner in that dinner leftovers make easy lunches.

Hamburger patties, a slice of ham, a chicken leg or two off yesterday's bird, deviled eggs,—all quick, easy, high protein, no carbohydrate. That spells "eat all you want." You can open a can of tuna or salmon or sardines or crabmeat. You can boil some frozen shrimp or a few frankfurters (make sure they are 100% meat).

Salami might have a carbo-cal or two per slice due to fillers but not enough to be concerned about. Tongue, liverwurst, pastrami, head cheese—the whole delicatessen is yours; including the cheese cases. There is only a trace of carbohydrate in most cheeses. Cottage cheese—the traditional starvation diet standby—is one of the highest in carbohydrate, with some ten carbo-cals in a five-ounce portion, 15 carbo-cals for the creamed variety.

Good news for cheese lovers

Pick your favorite cheese for lunch and eat all you want— American, Edam, Gruyere, Liederkranz, Limburger, Swiss, or Camembert. They are all excellent fat destroying foods.

Meat proteins

Of course, you can slice some of that turkey or turkey loaf, or cut a slab off that roast beef or leg of lamb or roast pork or ham or roast leg of veal. Dip in to the braised oxtail that you made for a couple of dinners, or the beef stew or lamb stew. Slice some flank steak kept for just such an occasion. Left-over cold fish is delicious.

If you can't make up your mind between two or three possibilities, have them all. You'll still lose weight.

Dinners

Come dinner time, when we are more willing to spend some time in preparation, the whole world of proteins opens up in a dazzling cavalcade of eating pleasure for even the most discriminating gourmet.

Liquor?

First a word about liquor. If you are accustomed to a martini or two before dinner, there are some 200 calories in one of these, but if it's a dry martini there are no carbo-cals to speak of. So, if you go on a starvation diet, forget the martinis. If you go on the no-carbohydrate or low-carbohydrate program, they remain, but easy on the vermouth.

Cheers.

On the OK list, too, are bourbon, rye, scotch, gin, vodka, and most brandies. Beer is out! Dry wines like claret or chablis have two carbo-cals per four ounce glass so they are permissible.

The main dinner dishes

On to main *dinner* dishes.

How many cuts of beef can you think of and how many ways to prepare each cut? From filet to flank, sirloin to stew, the varieties are endless. Add to these the number of cuts of lamb and pork and the ways to prepare them and you have menus enough for years of no repetition. Natural gravies, herbs, spices are splendid. Just don't thicken the sauce with flour or bread the cutlets.

Then, when you feel you've thought of everything, you'll remember braised oxtail and short rib stew and beef goulash and pigs knuckles and Swedish meatballs.

Do you think you know all there is to know about fish? How many ways can you prepare a salmon steak—broil, bake, poach? There are many more. Check any complete cookbook.

Fish dishes

How long has it been since you have had perch, cod, red snapper, halibut, haddock, flounder, or bluefish? Given a blindfold test, could you identify them by subtle flavor? How many more different fish can you think of? Did you remember to include turtle steaks, mussels, frogs' legs, eel?

Omit fish sticks, fish cakes and any kind of preparation involving flour or bread crumbs. Also, some of the more exotic ways of preparing lobster, for instance, include ingredients that add carbo-cals.

Poultry

Do you feel you know your poultry? Can you tell the difference between a squab and a cornish hen? Whether you like dark meat or light meat, eat all the turkey you want. Is goose fattening? Or duck? Not when you deprive it of carbohydrate hooks to hang on you. Quail, pheasant or just plain chicken, have yourself a ball with poultry—there's hardly a carbo-cal in sight.

Does all this sound attractive for your weight-losing campaign?

There you have it.

Do you think you'll ever be hungry while you are losing weight the high protein, fat destroyer way? Or will your taste buds ever be bored? Impossible.

There will be more types of foods that you will be able to enjoy—fruits, vegetables, desserts and beverages. But these will not be "eat all you want." Depending on whether you choose the *low*-carbohydrate or *no*-carbohydrate program, selection and quantities must be limited.

While you enjoy all these foods, you must remember to sidestep every lurking carbohydrate. Succumb to even just a few and all bets are off. Stay clear of them and you must lose weight.

There's almost no way not to.

Anatomy of a Fat Destroyer Food

Proteins, and even fats, are fat destroyer foods. Put them in the company of carbohydrates and they switch roles. *A protein or fat calorie, paired with a carbohydrate calorie, makes two fat producing calories.*

One carbohydrate calorie can change the life style of ten and even 20 protein calories. In other words if you are destroying your fat with 2,500 protein calories a day and you let 100 carbo-cals creep in, you will probably gain instead of lose.

You are better off eating 3,000 protein and fat calories. You will in all likelihood continue to lose. But let your carbo-cal guard down for just one beer and your fat destroyer foods are now geared to put the poundage on instead of take it off.

Proteins and fats are fat destroyer foods when there are no carbo-cals in sight. Ban them. Boycott them. Declare open war on them.

What I'm telling you is the truth.

What you hear on the food commercials or read on the labels or in the ads is sheer "sweet talk." Frozen waffles are not nourishing and "good for you." That sugary cereal that sounds good as well as tastes good is not as good as it sounds.

Yet this environmental bombardment is going to continue to attack your protein program.

You can reinforce your protein stance by understanding more about what proteins are and how they help to make you thin.

A Fact You Should Remember

Let me tell you one simple fact that speaks eloquently for proteins:

When you eat a diet of carbohydrates your metabolic rate goes down.

When you eat a diet of proteins your metabolic rate goes up.

This means you burn up more calories on proteins.

When you burn up more calories:

1. You store less as fat.
2. Or you can eat more without gaining weight.

The Role of Oxygen

It was Lavoisier, in the late eighteenth century, who showed that oxygen was used by the body to burn foods and create heat. He found that the consumption of food stepped up this process: more oxygen was consumed and more heat was lost by the body.

The Rubner Findings

About a century later, Rubner checked on the effect of different foods. First, he found that a man on a fast metabolized, or used-up, some 2,040 calories in 24 hours.

Then he put this man on a diet of 2,450 calories of sugar. The man metabolized 2,087, leaving over 350 calories stored in his body.

Next he put the man on the same calorie amount of meat. Now the man metabolized 2,566 calories, more than he took in.

This means on 2,450 calories of sugar the man was in a weight-gaining situation.

On the same 2,450 calories, but now meat (protein and fat), he was in a weight-losing situation.

Would you believe we've known this for a century now? Remember when family doctors wanted you to lose weight? What did they tell you to restrict?

"I want you to refrain from eating sweets and starches."

They knew what they were doing.

Let's say you were to eat just one fat destroyer food all day for a week. Now I'm not recommending this. You need different proteins—meats, fishes, cheeses, eggs, poultry—to give your body an assortment of amino acids, minerals, vitamins and other nutrients often needed in only trace amounts but nevertheless critical.

But let's say you chose chopped sirloin. You ate a hefty quarter-pound for breakfast, half-pound for lunch and three-quarters of a pound for dinner. That's one and one-half pounds at about 1,650 prote-cals per pound or 2,475 for the day.

Calories down the Drain

This would be close to the allotment in the Rubner experiments. Does this mean that you would have weight loss advantage of only about one hundred calories (2,566 - 2,475 = 91)? Since one pound is about 3,500 calories, you would lose only one pound a month, if that.

Actually, you lose faster on the all-protein diet because other metabolic changes occur, besides that discovered by Rubner.

Calories go down the drain when you eat proteins alone. Urea and other waste products of protein metabolism are excreted by the body without being burned or stored.

It's just as if protein fuel was not burned efficiently. You don't have to be concerned about every protein calorie going into energy or fat storage. Unlike carbohydrate calories, protein calories get wasted—turned into waste.

Did you ever notice that sometimes your urine seems thicker, more viscous and yellow than other times? And did you ever notice that sometimes your excrement floats in the toilet bowl while other times it sinks? Protein calories encourage heavier waste.

We can excrete lightweight or heavyweight material. We can also excrete low-calorie or high-calorie material. Protein calories encourage higher calorie waste.

Also, when we drink non-caloric water, tea or coffee, we can absorb the liquid or excrete it. Protein programs encourage less absorption of water, more excretion of it.

Roman food orgies were punctuated by massage sessions. The intestines were worked to move the material along and accelerate its eventual removal from the body. In this way, the revelers would make room more quickly for the gluttony to follow. In a way, high-protein foods move themselves along and out. If we were a factory instead of a body, protein would be an inefficient fuel to burn.

Recommended fuel for factories where every calorie counts— carbohydrates.

You Can Stay Fat If You Want to

Recently, the National Association to Aid Fat Americans was formed. When I heard about it, I wondered whether their aid was directed at exposing the insidiousness of the carbohydrate and educating their members about fat destroying proteins.

Instead, I found that this is a group dedicated to making fat people more at ease about being fat. "Fat is beautiful," they say. "If dieting has proved unsuccessful, why feel pressured to diet any more?"

I don't know how this strikes you. But here's how it strikes me. Sure, you have the freedom to choose obesity if you want it. But you better darn well know what you're getting into when you get into a fat body.

It would be nice, from Mr. Big's point of view, to have him in demand by women. Or for Miss Big to be stared at in her bikini in admiration rather than disbelief.

But it's not going to happen in America. Even in Hawaii, where bigness has been a sign of royal blood, the corpulent Hawaiian men and women are yielding to the lither Polynesian types.

Who Is "Mr. Big"?

It would be nice for Mr. Big to be respected by top executives and make it to the top himself. But this does not happen in America, either. A survey by a large personnel agency shows that of the executives in the $25,000 to $50,000 bracket only 10 percent are overweight, compared to 35 percent under $20,000.

There seems to be an appreciation of tall thin people, as opposed to short fat ones, right from the word "go." It has been found that, all else being equal, teachers give better marks to the taller, thinner youngsters. Some college admission policies systematically reject overweight applicants.

Even doctors have been found to discriminate against overweight patients. A Duke University survey of physicians' attitudes revealed such comments as "ugly," "awkward," "weak-willed" recorded for the corpulent ones.

Heavy eater, heavy drinker, heavy smoker—it doesn't seem to matter what your "bag" is—excessive anything takes years off your life expectancy.

In the case of excessive eating and its attendant bulges, even 10 percent overweight people are biting off what they might rather eschew: tendency to heart disease, gall stones, and diabetes mellitus. They are prone to cardiovascular and renal diseases which affect the heart, blood vessels and kidneys.

Now I know you don't want to hear this. Your subconscious, which has been programmed to eat the way that you now eat, is rebelling and sending you sly thoughts of putting the book down for awhile.

Well, why don't you put the book down for a minute or two and have a talk with "George." Tell your subconscious that all is well. On this diet of high protein foods you will be able to continue to eat all you want—of the right foods. Put "George" at ease. Then read on and convince yourself that the price of carbohydrates is too high.

You Pay a Price for Every
Excess Pound of Fat

Man has many carry-overs from his primitive days. Anxiety, formerly directed at an approaching danger and now directed at business problems, still triggers the acid secretions once necessary for efficient flight but now only good for ulcer-producing. Fear that made ancient man's hair stand on end—and which still gives us that creepy feeling in our scalp—did so for a purpose: to make him appear bigger and more fearsome to his enemy.

At one time man—like the camel—stored fat on his back as protection against lean and hungry days. This is still visible among some African tribes. But today, whether stored on the back or front, fat is a sign of diet imbalance.

And imbalance leads to a fall.

How the Insurance Companies Figure Fat

There is a rule of thumb that is popular in insurance circles. It says that a person who is 50 years of age and 50 pounds overweight has 50 percent less life expectancy.

This means that at 50, a man of normal weight can expect to live 18 more years. But a man with 50 pounds of extra baggage can expect to live only nine more years.

For a woman of 50 it means she can expect to live 20 more years if she is of normal weight but if she it toting 50 extra pounds, it looks more like only ten years to go.

It isn't always just "curtains." There can be years of suffering for seriously overweight people. Here is what can be on the menu for some people who choose to be fat.

The Hidden Menace of Eating for Satisfaction

You say you are "built for comfort not for speed," but do you call the gnawing pain of arthritis comfortable? About all you can say for the various forms of arthritis is that they are only crippling, not killing. Joints gradually become immobilized so that movement is excruciating. For some arthritics, even lying still in bed is painful. Seriously overweight people are candidates for this "living hell."

Also in the medical menu for Humpty-Dumpty is diabetes. This is a carbohydrate-related metabolic disorder in which the ability to oxidize these villains is lost to a degree. This happens when the pancreas can no longer produce enough of the hormone called insulin. Thirst, hunger and weakness are the usual symptoms, with sugar in the urine as a testable symptom. Diabetics must give themselves insulin shots by needle daily at the risk of otherwise going into a condition of shock or even coma.

Not very appetizing is it? Nor are inflammation of the gall bladder, cirrhosis of the liver, high blood pressure or varicose veins.

Fat people get hernias more often because of the strain of extra weight on tendons. Furthermore, they make poor surgical patients. It is difficult enough for a surgeon to get to an appendix or gall bladder, but to cut through layers of blubber increases the hazards. These operations are fatal four times more frequently for fat people.

If you are seriously overweight you are:

- More prone to having accidents.
- Less virile and sexually potent.
- Less fertile.
- More likely to have pregnancy complications.
- Less resistant to infectious diseases.

It all adds up to a very definite price spelled out in years of life per pound of excess weight.

I have prepared a table expressing this exorbitant price. It is based on actuarial tables. Look it over. The years of life lost will be *your* years. See chart on "Cost of Overweight Pounds in YEARS OF LIFE LOST" on p. 55.

The New Deal Possible for You—The Easy Path

It's easy to understand that there can be a National Association to Aid Fat Americans. They need help. But not help to live with their round shape; help to get rid of it.

The path is no longer strewn with melba toast and carrot sticks.

There is no longer any need to be hungry, to fail, to feel remorse, to begin over, to be hungry, to fail again.

Rather, it is an easy path, strewn with lamb chops and oysters Rockefeller.

Hunger is out. Failure is out.

You can go only one way and that is toward your attractive, slender, vital self.

Let's drink to a longer, healthier life for a slender you. How about a scotch on the rocks? You can have it without wondering about your weight or this book's campaign for weight-losing.

Skol.

Cost of Overweight Pounds in YEARS OF LIFE LOST

MEN

Age	Up to 50 lbs.*	50 to 100 lbs.*	Over 100 lbs.*
40	10	20	30
50	9	15	18
60	8	10	11
70	5	7	8

WOMEN

Age	Up to 30 lbs.*	30 to 70 lbs.*	Over 70 lbs.*
40	7	15	22
50	6	14	20
60	4	9	13
70	3	7	9

*The years lost are less when weight has not persisted as many years.

HOW TO FEED YOUR BODY BETTER,
NOT WORSE, TO LOSE WEIGHT

I do not cringe at the number of pompous voices that will hit back at me to protest the basic concept of eating all you want and still losing weight.

But I'll be glad to take the lumps as long as my slenderizing clients continue to lose theirs.

They are still not ready even to investigate this program. But one day these nutritionists will say, "We knew it all along!"

The more you—the reader who wishes to lose weight and stay slim—know about foods and their effects on your body, the more you will see the connection between food manufacturers and nutritionists. They are a team, forced by the economics of the food industry to work together. This chapter gets into specifics of my campaign.

Food Advertising's Impact on You

The farmer or rancher cannot afford to employ a nutritionist to tell you about the value of his fresh, natural product. But the manufacturer of a bread or a cereal or some other kind of packaged, processed food is producing a nationally-sold item and can profit by employing a university nutritionist as a consultant to praise his product.

He can also buy advertising in your local newspaper, in magazines, on radio, and on television. Begin, today, to read and listen to these ads and commercials in a new way.

Let me explain this way. There's a hotel in a famous resort. It is not in the center of things, so to compensate its guests for this inconvenience it runs a shuttle bus back and forth free of charge. On the bus in big letters is the name of the hotel and this plug: "Closest to the fun!"

Ads for processed foods often go this same route. They take their weakness and call it a strength. They don't tell you that the food processor is very efficient in removing the "live" nutrients so the shelf life will be longer. They just try to portray in their ads as their strength what they're really missing: nutrition. And they show pictures of healthy young children eating their denatured carbohydrate that has been sugared to taste better, preserved with chemicals to last longer, and artificially colored to look better.

Can you imagine your body's disappointment after it has gone to the trouble of biting, chewing, swallowing, and digesting to find nary a protein, mineral or vitamin to nourish it.

"Fooled again," says your body. "It's only carbohydrate. Store this stuff in the buttocks." How sadly true it is!

The Junk that Pulls the Wool over Your Eyes and the Fat over Your Body

Look at food ads a new way. Question what they proclaim. Suspect that what they say is their strength is more likely their weakness.

Food processors are churning out tons of non-nutritive foods and beverages daily. They are usually high in fat-producing carbo-cals, and high in preservative chemicals, some of which are suspect as the causes of cancer and birth defects.

They sell these tons of junk by glamorizing it as food. Funk and Wagnall's dictionary defines food as "That which is eaten or drunk or absorbed for the growth and repair of organisms and the maintenance of life; nourishment; nutriment; aliment."

Dogs and cats, rats and mice die if fed exclusively on this factory goo sold to humans as food. It is certainly not fit for human consumption and the only reason that humans survive it is that there are still some of nature's products around.

I like profits. I am a proponent of the profit system. But it has checks and balances. Management cannot exploit labor for more profit. It needs another internal check or balance: food factories should not be permitted to make more profit by providing less nutrition.

To add insult to injury, the vested interests in fabricated foods dare to attack the fledgling health food movement as faddist. I have no ax to grind for organic foods or so-called health foods. But it is this movement that has opened our eyes to what is happening to our food.

If farmers were not trying to improve their yield with chemical fertilizers, chemical sprays, and other devices such as keeping lights on all night to encourage egg laying, their products might taste better—fruits and vegetables would have the flavor they do in European countries, poultry would be less antiseptic and bland to the palate, tomatoes would be deep red with juice.

If food processors would pay as much attention to nutrition as they do to attrition and spoilage, there would be no health food industry to attack.

I would certainly favor health foods over the carbohydrate garbage that is foisted on us under the guise of nutrition. If you had only two sources of food—a health food store or a store with only processed foods—which one would you pick? I don't think there is any doubt that you'd live longer the health food way.

Fortunately, we don't have to go to either extreme. We have a greater choice to consider.

Guidelines for Feeling Great
As You Lose Weight

For your continued good health, for faster weight loss, for successful maintenance of your slim profile, for better nutrition, I recommend that you adopt the following priorities:

Proteins over fats and carbohydrates.
Fats over carbohydrates.

Fresh meats over frozen.

Lightly cooked meats over well done.

Natural meats (if you can find them) over those forced with hormones and other unnatural methods.

Meats in the natural state over canned meats, sausages, wursts, etc.

Fresh fruits and vegetables over canned or packaged or frozen.

Frozen fruits and vegetables over canned or packaged.

Raw fruits and vegetables over cooked.

Local fruits and vegetables over those transported over long distances.

Organic fruits and vegetables over those that have been chemically fertilized and sprayed.

Whole grains over enriched and denatured grains.

Enriched grains over denatured grains.

Everyone of these priorities is aimed at making your metabolic processes work at highest efficiency. You can get by with less. We are all getting by with less. But the higher you are able to adhere to this list of priorities, the better your body will feel as you lose pound after pound.

My aim is to make you feel wonderful while you lose and while you maintain your proper weight. The better you feel losing weight and staying slim, the less likely you'll want to return to those old sweet and starchy days.

The Most Permissive Diet Ever to Drop Pounds Off People

You would lose weight and be bursting with health if you observed the above priorities.

However, even if you could only observe several of them strictly, you would also lose weight.

Let me put it this way:

Here is a "Free Diet"—Eat any food, drink any liquid EXCEPT

- No food or liquid that contains flour, starch, or sugar.
- Limit alcohol to two ounces daily of distilled spirits or six ounces daily of dry wine.

You will lose weight on this diet, if you are excessively fat-burdened, say 30 or more pounds overweight.

Soon you will stop losing weight, but you will begin again if you tighten up on your priorities.

Here is how to start the weight loss moving again when it slows up:

- Exercise protein priority over other foods.
- Make other calories count nutrition-wise by buying local, buying fresh, cooking less.

A difficult case to handle—
the average housewife

Molly was a difficult case. She almost never ate a sitdown meal. Her intake of food consisted of the leftovers of her childrens' breakfast and lunch, her "tasting" while she was making dinner and a quart of ice cream late at night when no one was looking.

Over the years, she had joined numerous weight-losing organizations, had spent three years in psychotherapy, and had dieted strenuously. She had managed, through these efforts, to lose about 200 pounds. Unfortunately, she had also managed to gain about 260 pounds, so that she was 60 pounds heavier than the 140 pounds she had weighed when she first decided to diet, 15 years ago.

I instructed her not to diet,—just keep doing what she was doing. But . . . she must write everything down.

She returned a week later with a list which, when analyzed, ran less than 15 percent protein. Over the next month, she was taught to select high protein foods and was encouraged to continue writing down what she ate.

She brought the protein content up to a weight-losing level by excluding all carbohydrates except vegetables, salads and fruit and by allowing herself only one portion each of these carbohydrates daily. She ate freely of all meat, fish, poultry, cheese and eggs.

She lost weight very satisfactorily. The last I heard she was below 140 and still losing. As a fortuitous by-product, she found time for a sit-down breakfast, lunch, and dinner.

There are a number of diets in the pages ahead. This is the most permissive. The last is the most restrictive.

How to Get Your Weight
Losing Program Going

It is best to start with the most permissive and check results. If you've fifty pounds of excess baggage, there's no need of going on the same tight calorie budget as a model with three stubborn pounds to get rid of.

The Free Diet

One woman who went on this Free Diet began to gain weight instead of losing it. About the only thing she had given up when she went on the diet was her liquor. She was used to a few shots around lunchtime and a few more in the evening. Now she had taken to drinking huge volumes of orange juice. She confessed she went through two six-ounce cans of frozen juice a day—actually 48 ounces of juice, or nearly 700 calories a day, most of them carbo-cals.

She was better off weight-wise on the other "juice."

There is sugar in orange juice.

There is starch in green peas.

True, these are natural sugars and as such provide you with nutritive benefits in exchange for calories, more than one can say for that refined white stuff.

But you have to be realistic on this Free Diet. All you eliminate is sugar and starch. You must be conscientious about doing this. Take this away from the Free Diet and it isn't going to take anything away from you.

How a fat man handled his problem

Tony is a case in point. Tony's problem was that he never had access to the right food when he needed it. He could not stand breakfast, although he admitted he enjoyed breakfast on weekends and when he was on vacation. He never had time to go out for lunch and would send out for a sandwich and a coke from a not-too-modern diner which was situated up the block from his warehouse. He worked late almost every night and would "grab something" whenever he could. When he got home, he would relax, which to him meant—eat.

In fact, very often he would buy a large pizza on the way home and that, with two cans of beer and a half of an apple pie, was his favorite supper. He also liked spaghetti and had bragged he could consume four helpings without hardly taking a breath.

Tony was grotesque. I could not weigh him. My scales had a maximum of 400 pounds. When he stood on the scale the arm flew up and I knew that he weighed considerably more, but I had no way of telling how much more.

Tony's real problem

The interesting thing about Tony was that 80 percent of his daily intake was eaten almost immediately before going to bed, a time when he expended little energy and therefore few calories. It was all stored as fat. "Often," he stated proudly "I do not touch a thing all day."

I explained to him the difficulty of maintaining weight in that manner. I asked him how he would like to lose weight on six meals a day instead of gaining weight on one meal a day. He took me up on this. I handed him a copy of our Miracle Diet book[1], and he promised to read it before our next visit. Then our work began.

He was encouraged to feed his appetite starting from the morning with a healthy serving of eggs and bacon or ham or sausages.

The same diner that sent up the sandwiches now sent up what was inside the sandwiches,—chicken salad, egg salad, shrimp salad, pot roast, turkey and so on but without the bread, just lettuce and tomato.

Tony also was instructed to eat dinner at a reasonable time and to travel to one of several good restaurants, which were within ten minutes of his office, where he could take his choice from an abundant menu of steaks, chops and lobsters or any other meat, fish or fowl dish that hit his fancy. He was also encouraged to have a light second breakfast, lunch, or dinner if the mood struck him.

---

[1] *The Miracle Diet,* Petrie and Stone, West Nyack, N.Y.: Parker Publishing Company.

For the time being, he was not to follow any precise diet but under no circumstances was he to eat any food that contained either starch or sugar. He could eat any kind of meat, fish, poultry, cheese, eggs, salads, vegetables, fruits, and fats that he wanted.

I saw him each week after he started on this Free Diet. Each week we would watch the scale to see if the arm would move. At the fourth week it did, pointing to 398 pounds. We calculated by his change in belt size that he had probably lost 40 pounds in those four weeks but we will never be sure. In any case, he is continuing to lose weight very nicely and eventually, when the weight loss stops, Tony will be ready to move to a somewhat more restricted diet.

Starch in Foods

There is no sugar or starch in meat, eggs, poultry, fish or cheese. Eat all you want, provided that your preparation includes no bread crumbs, cornstarch or sweetenings.

Some vegetables are very starchy. Potatoes are the classic example.

Some fruits and melons are very sweet, like watermelon, and starchy, like bananas.

Steer a wide berth around these types if you want to avoid a wide girth.

A Helpful Table to Guide You

To help you know which fruits and vegetables are low in sugar and starch, a table appears in the center section of this book. It shows the total calories for typical measurements of just about every type of food you can think of.

But it shows much more. It shows the percentage of protein in each food. And then it shows the protein, fat, and carbohydrate calories in each food.

It is this last column—the carbohydrate calories—that can be a valuable guide to you on the Free Diet.

If you look now at the vegetable section of this list and let your eye run down the right hand column, you will see carbohydrate calories exceeding the hundred mark for such vegetables as potatoes, lentils, lima beans, corn. These are foods with starch in them—to be avoided with a vengeance.

Even those under the hundred should be side-stepped wherever possible, especially when they exceed 50 carbo-cals.

Under 50 carbo-cals are such delicious vegetables as broccoli, cabbage, carrots, leeks, peppers, tomatoes, some types of squash, and all types of greens.

As you glance along that left-hand column, you will also see a number of vegetables under ten carbo-cals. They are mostly greens but very valuable to your body as you lose weight. Note these. Check those with which you are familiar and which you enjoy. Put several on your next shopping list.

Spanish onions, green scallions, mushrooms, asparagus, cabbage, egg plant, leeks, celery, spinach, cucumbers—these are just a few of the vegetables you can eat on the Free Diet, knowing without a shadow of a doubt that you have made a starch-free, sugar-free choice.

As to fruits, a glance down the right-hand column in that category shows that these run higher in carbo-cals than vegetables. That is, the fruits lowest in carbo-cals are still higher in carbo-cals than the greens.

The best you can do in fruits is to stay clear of canned and frozen varieties, most of which are canned in syrup or frozen with sugar added.

Lean *toward* grapefruit, cantaloupe, berries and *away* from bananas, watermelon, and dried fruits.

This is a Free Diet so eat whatever fruit you want. An apple, pear, peach, or plum is not going to undercut your weight loss.

The Free Diet can be the answer for many overweight people. The elimination of the bulk of sweets and starches can do the trick.

However, others may have to bear down harder on these sweets and starches.

How We Continue to Make Deposits in Our Calorie Bank

Nutritionists probably have more to learn about food and human metabolism than they already know, but there are some valuable facts about proteins, carbohydrates, and fats that have been established.

The daddy of American nutritionists was W.O. Atwater who did extensive laboratory work to determine the energy equivalents of the various classes of foods. He found that basically:

> One gram of protein = four calories
> One gram of carbohydrate = four calories
> One gram of fat = nine calories

Since one ounce equals 28.35 grams:

> One ounce of protein = 113 calories
> One ounce of carbohydrate = 113 calories
> One ounce of fat = 255 calories

So, ounce for ounce, proteins and carbohydrates give us the same number of calories. But we no longer fall into the traditionalists' trap that a calorie is a calorie.

We know that one carbo-cal is far more dangerous than one prote-cal. One ounce of carbohydrate is far more fattening than one ounce of protein.

Calorie-Burning Methods

Here is another set of interesting facts. How many calories do you burn jogging, swimming, or just plain walking?

These have been determined for a number of activities, based on your weight. It is necessary to tie the calories consumed per hour to the weight of the person doing the activity because, obviously, a heavy person exerts more energy than a light person in moving himself from one point to another.

Here are the calories consumed per hour by a one-hundred pound person and a two-hundred pound person. If you are in between, you can figure the proportionate amount that applies to you.

CALORIES EXPENDED PER HOUR

	100 Lb. Person	200 Lb. Person
Sleeping	40	80
Sitting	60	120
Standing	60	120
Walking slowly	130	260

CALORIES EXPENDED PER HOUR (*cont.*)

	100 Lb. Person	200 Lb. Person
Walking moderately fast	190	380
Bicycling	280	560
Jogging	360	720
Exercising strenuously	380	760
Running very fast	470	940
Swimming	475	950

If you weigh 150 pounds, you expend 540 calories an hour jogging. Since one pound of human fat is considered to be equivalent to 3,500 calories, you would have to jog for over six hours to lose one pound of "pudge." And what do you think even one hour of jogging does to your appetite?

If you weigh 150 pounds, you expend about 700 calories an hour swimming. To exact your pound of flesh, it would take five hours in the water providing you don't waste time floating to catch your breath.

Exercise is not the answer to weight loss. Exercise cannot be sustained long enough. On the other hand, active people burn more calories than those with sedentary life styles. They can eat more and not show it. Conversely, when you step up your daily working or living activities, you might lose weight without changing your eating habits.

A secretary quits to take a job with the town as a meter maid. She spends 130 calories an hour eight hours a day instead of her former 60 calories an hour sitting, or a total extra expenditure of 560 calories. If she works five and one half days a week in her first month, she could lose three pounds,—providing she doesn't make an extra stop at the corner luncheonette each afternoon.

A foreman in an assembly plant is promoted to a desk job. This takes about 1,000 calories less per day. That's equivalent to a large meal. Does he give up dinner? Hardly. He keeps eating as before, because its a habit, and might even add a couple of martinis before lunch just to keep up with his executive-type colleagues.

More money from the corporation, and more corporation on him.

Moral: it takes a change in eating habits, not working or exercising habits to change weight.

We learn another lesson from the activity calorie expended table. Look at the calories expended sleeping. A 150-pound person uses up 480 during an eight-hour night. Yet, just before retiring, that person can consume for dinner, television snacks and a night cap three times that much.

Where does it go? Take a look in the mirror.

Did you make a deposit in your calorie bank last night?

Why a High Protein Breakfast Takes More Weight off You Than No Breakfast at All

Portrait of an overweight person: "I don't eat breakfast—I'm just not hungry—lunch is a quick bite—sometimes skip even that—a drink or two before dinner—by that time I'm hungry and dig in—if there are leftovers, I knock them off before midnight."

You don't lose weight by depriving yourself of a meal. You make up for it later.

In fact, you *more* than make up for it later!

The first meal of the day is very important in weight control. When you arise, your blood sugar is at a normal level. If you don't eat, you reduce your blood sugar level. This creates hunger. When you are hungry, you eat more. Then you are likely to experience cycles of hunger and over-eating the rest of the day.

Now let's say you eat breakfast. But you eat a carbohydrate breakfast: Orange juice, English muffin and coffee. Or a bowl of sugar-added "tasties."

Most carbohydrate foods are out of your stomach in two hours.

Carbohydrates enter your bloodstream as blood sugar quite fast. A big carbohydrate dose might trigger the fat-converting process.

On the other hand, proteins take an average of four hours to clear your stomach. During this period, you are not likely to feel hungry, and your bloodstream is getting a slow but steady supply of energy, with no need for your body to activate its fat-storing process.

Moral: High protein breakfasts "stick to your ribs" for a few hours instead of to your waist for a few years.

The Free Diet Can Work Miracles
for Your Weight Losing Campaign

Imagine eating all you want, never counting calories, merely side-stepping sweets and starches—and dropping pound after pound!

It sounds too good to be true. But it is true and it has lost tons for my clients.

The best part of the Free Diet is that, since it is not really a diet in the restrictive sense, there is no getting off or ending it. So you never gain back the weight you lose.

A "Big" Man's Experience
With Free Diet

The Free Diet often works where far more stringent methods fail. Jack had what the weight tables describe as a large frame. He was tall, 6'4", and up to age 40 was able to eat exactly what he felt like eating, without gaining an ounce.

He was very active, played football, basketball and regularly jogged through the park.

Coincidentally, with his fortieth birthday he married, changed jobs and gradually became less physically active. He continued to eat as he always ate. His favorites were spaghetti, steak and potatoes, apple pie and midnight snacks. Within six months, his bathroom scale showed he had gained 35 pounds.

Realizing that his weight gain was mainly due to decreased physical activity, he attempted to return to his sports but found that for one reason or another his new life simply did not give him the time.

Jack tried several diets but felt hungry on all of them. Appetite-depressant pills created irritability. They were also disruptive in his office and family relationships. The result was a net gain instead of a net loss. He gradually became 50 pounds overweight.

When Jack went on the Free Diet, he found that the foods permitted were completely satisfying to him. They allowed him to eat at home, socially, and at business meetings without feeling deprived or frustrated. His weight declined gradually to approximately ten pounds above his normal weight. He was not willing to eat less to lose this slight excess. However, it really did not matter since on his 6'4" frame ten pounds were insignificant. What was significant was that he was willing to stay on the Free Diet as a maintenance diet. And the 40 pounds he lost, stayed lost.

A Case History of an Introverted Female

Danni had been a plump little girl. Later, she had been a fat little adolescent, an overweight young woman and at 30, she was now, you guessed it, flabby. Danni's mother, with whom she still lived, screamed, threatened, and cajoled for almost every day of Danni's life. Danni had never dated, had never dared to wear a bathing suit, and had never owned a dress that looked decent on her.

As a teenager, she had tried amphetamines to drop pounds, but they had made her deathly ill. Later, in desperation, she tried them again—this time finishing up in the hospital for 11 weeks. While lying on her back in the hospital enjoying both the hospital's fare and her mother's sympathy cakes, Danni gained 20 more pounds.

Danni was a food addict. If a diet allowed her one slice of bread, it was like offering one ounce of whiskey to an alcoholic. Goodbye, loaf. Diet recipes which made food look and taste more appetizing with less calories were of no use to her for her reasoning was that as this delicious food was low-caloried she could eat four times as much of it.

This deception is practiced fairly universally amongst dieters. Many "diet" foods on the market are only a few calories less than the same foods in their regular state. The dieters then become permissive, eat of these foods freely, and in the end ingest more calories than they would have by purchasing the regular foods.

Danni began with me on the Free Diet. Her excessive poundage began to drop off like the wax from a burning candle. She became enthusiastic about this new kind of a diet and I continuously encouraged her. Her mother, for some reason, did not cooperate. She would buy Danni's old, fattening foods at the supermarket and display them temptingly in the house. Twice her mother called me and complained that Danni was losing weight too fast and it was not good for her. I was too angry to argue and referred her to Danni's physician. Somehow, I felt, the mother needed to have the fat on Danni just to be able to continue to "bug" and boss her.

As the weight kept pouring off her, Danni became aware that men were paying attention to her. One tried to make a date with her. In fact, he eventually did. It was her only date and she married him.

After awhile, Danni's weight approached normal and her weight loss stopped. The permissive foods on the Free Diet were too much to bring her down to her normal weight of about 120 pounds, but some minor adjustment on quantities eventually slipped her into a size eight.

Danni, the plump baby, the fat adolescent and overweight young woman is now a slender wife. I phoned her recently to update the record. She is putting back a little weight now. But that's all right because in a few months she is going to have a baby.

The Weight Problem of a Professional Man and How It Was Solved

Sol, by profession a doctor of dentistry, was getting paunchy. Sol stood six feet tall. His black hair was attractively speckled with gray and as a sign of the times, he had sprouted a proud, jet black, semi-handlebar moustache. Recently divorced, he was a prize target of the unmarried females for miles around.

Always meticulous in his personal appearance, he had a full and extensive wardrobe but it was gradually producing tight and uncomfortable pressures around his middle. Since his divorce he ate out a great deal, taking his dates to the finest restaurants, and eating much more than when he was married. Also he traveled more, completing trips to Greece and to a dental convention in Australia. He was eating his way around the world and getting rounder himself.

However, Sol was not diet-minded. He was gourmet food-minded. He enjoyed living well. He prided himself on his impeccable taste in clothes, food, and women. The Free Diet was made to order for him.

On it, Sol began to enjoy steaks and lobsters, Long Island duck, and salads heaped high with Roquefort dressing. He never missed the bread, rolls, potatoes, and desserts. He now fits comfortably into his clothing because his radius has diminished. Meanwhile, the radius of female interest has spread considerably.

The more wisdom you put into your dining in the Free Diet, the more likely you can stay with it and not have to go on a more restrictive program.

Exercise these priorities spelled out earlier in this chapter. Stay with the highest protein foods, also the highest mineral- and vitamin-content foods. Become nutrition-conscious.

Also, eat breakfast; don't skip this important meal.

Eat as frequently as you wish, keeping meals moderate. A large meal triggers the body's fat-storing mechanisms. Two smaller meals, properly spaced, feed your body with fuel as needed.

Try to eat more during the day, less late in the day. Big dinners or late snacks, coming when little fuel will be needed while you're asleep, are sure ways to compel the body to store that fuel as unwanted fat.

Have a Kitchen Cleaning Party
to Begin Your Free Diet

Let's get started.

Let's begin to slim down to our best, most attractive, healthful weight.

No, not today. Tomorrow.

If this sounds like the typical dieter procrastinating, wait. There's a method in my mimicry.

You need to make some preparations for this Free Diet. Can you guess what's coming? You need to get a broom and sweep your house clean of dirty, old carbohydrates.

Get your friends in to help. Have a Cala-bash. Let them go through your cupboards and refrigerator and grab anything with sugar, flour, or starch in it.

Make fudge. Serve all that frozen cake. Finish off the bar and sweet wine. Clean out the cookie jar.

Cook the frozen lima beans and other starchy vegetables. Put them on a buffet. Let the ladies help you concoct carbohydrate casseroles with the potatoes, peas, and such still in your vegetable inventory. Make Boston baked beans with cans on the shelf. Let your friends dig out the carbohydrate stuff and come up with ideas for cooking and serving.

Give door prizes: two pounds of sugar, three pounds of flour, a half used jar of orange marmalade, a package of marshmallows, a jumbo box of wheat flakes, what's left of a package of corn starch, etc.

Can you join them in the eating part? Sure you can. Stuff yourself. Did they make a pizza? Wolf it down. Try every casserole. Have the ice cream and melt some of the fudge over it.

Even when you are full, force yourself to have another piece of cake, another cookie.

The hidden message

Begin to feel the sickening, bloating effects of sweets and starches. It may take you a day or two or three to burn off those miserable, fattening carbo-cals, but if they make you begin to detest them, it's worth it.

Maybe your friends will get the message, too. It may change their life. Don't preach to them, or try to talk them into doing what you are about to do.

Just let them celebrate with you. Let them toast your forthcoming slender self, your freedom from the tyranny of the carbo-cal. Leave this book lying on a table. Perhaps, as they say their goodnights after a fun evening, and return home with a loaf of white bread under their arm, they'll give it some second thoughts.

Meanwhile: you are invited to another party starting the next morning at breakfast time. Come as you are. It is a High Protein Party. It is going to go on and on. You'll have a ball.

RSVP.

4

YOU WILL BE EATING WELL ON THE
FAT DESTROYER HIGH PROTEIN DIET

How a Slim Clothes Model Won Her Battle

Linda was married on her twentieth birthday and everyone agreed that she was a most beautiful bride. She had spent two years as a model for a New York couturier house, and as she walked down the aisle, you could tell Linda was playing her good looks to the hilt.

Eight years and three babies later, Linda was ushered into my office. She sat down without a word and began to cry. "You are my last hope," she sobbed, and gradually began to unfold her tale of how she had gained 40 pounds since her wedding day.

She had never had to worry about her weight. By nature she was not a big eater and rarely ate fattening foods. During her first pregnancy, she had put on 30 pounds. After her child was born, she still retained eight pounds, which somehow she could not seem to get off. The births of her second and third children were responsible for an additional 20 pounds.

Now she could not eat as haphazardly as she had done before her marriage. Although she claimed that she ate "carefully," her weight was climbing slowly but steadily.

Her fattening menu

Her daily menu ran something like this:

Breakfast: Orange juice, coffee and a slice of toast with marmalade.
Lunch: A sandwich of some kind and a glass or two of juice, usually apple or pineapple.
5:00 p.m. Coffee Break: A corn or bran muffin or a toasted English muffin and coffee.
Dinner: A meat, fish or poultry dish with salad and vegetable and for dessert most often fruit, but occasionally a small piece of cake or pie.
Late Snack: Some raw or canned fruit and cottage cheese.

What her menu did to her

Let's examine this diet more carefully. What is its protein, carbohydrate and fat content? Breakfast, the orange juice is greater than 90 percent carbohydrate and so is the marmalade. The toast is about 80 percent carbohydrate. Lunch contained some protein in the form of meat, fish or poultry in the sandwich; the rest—the bread, lettuce and tomato—are 80 percent carbohydrate.

The late afternoon muffin is about as bad. The vegetable, salad and fruit at dinner time are high carbohydrates. For example, an innocent orange is 85 percent carbohydrate, and juices almost 100 percent. Her total intake of calories was almost entirely carbohydrate.

Her total food intake for the day would be considered normal for most people. It would not cause a weight gain in Linda except for one thing: carbo-cals. As in the case of thousands of frustrated dieters, Linda's protein intake was far too low for her to lose weight.

How her menu was adjusted

I adjusted her menus with her. We eliminated most of the carbohydrate intake substituting protein in its place. She gave up nothing. Yet, she was able to lose weight. She lost four of those 40 pounds the very first week. The rate of loss tapered off but so did she. In three months she looked great again.

Years later, I checked on Linda. She has remained slender and said she was considering doing TV commercials. You have heard of models having to "starve" themselves to be models. Now you surely have a different concept as to how models can "eat for their jobs."

The Switch to Protein Is Easy to Make

Switching to proteins is easy. We seem to consider the meat part of any meal as the focal point of that meal.

Suppose I asked you to become a vegetarian to lose weight. Nine out of ten people would balk. They would feel that they were giving up the backbone of their meals.

We seem to have a natural inclination to include meat, fish, poultry, cheese, or eggs in every meal. This must have something to do with protein being the prime body building food as well as the prime fat destroying food. Our natural intuition moves toward protein foods.

I am not asking you to become a vegetarian. Nor am I asking you to become a meatarian. I am asking you to replace sweets, flours, and starches with meat or other proteins.

When you destroy fat this way, you are on a balanced diet. Perhaps it is not balanced in the eyes of the Delicious Baking Company or the Delightful Cereal Company—and their paid nutritional consultants—but it is balanced in the eyes of our grandparents and their grandparents.

The carbohydrate trap

In this generation of manufacturing progress, the competition to build a better carbohydrate trap has flooded supermarket shelves with so many quick and easy "foods" vying for our budget dollar that their hue and cry drowns out the gentle pull of lamb chops and turnip greens.

Take a child to the supermarket and he reaches out to the clowns on the cereal boxes as you go by, and to the cookies, candies, and cakes. He ogles at see-through boxes showing the cones, creamsickles, and other carbohydrate confections.

But does he see any cartoons on the legs of lamb? Does he reach out for the chicken, veal, or beef? Is he fascinated by the red, orange, and yellow designs on packages of asparagus or watercress?

We have permitted this carbohydrate bombardment to unbalance our diets. If you have any doubt about this, squeeze the rolls of fat on your abdomen, hips, and thighs. Feel that hanging stuff on your rump, ribs, and arms.

Most of it came from foods invented in the last 50 years.

These foods have *un*balanced our diet.

A billion-dollar food processing industry has now spawned a billion-dollar diet food and weight reducing industry.

One hand fattens the other.

Can Nature's Foods Compare with Processed Foods?

At the University of California in Santa Cruz, there is a health food cafeteria called the Whole Earth Restaurant. Staffed by ten students, the restaurant features an open kitchen where people can move around freely and talk to the cooks. This kitchen is a living class in natural foods and how to prepare them without destroying their natural flavors and nutrients.

A previous manager of this restaurant is Mrs. Sharon Cadwallader, co-author with Judi Ohr of the *Whole Earth Cookbook,* in which she strikes back at food processors in behalf of Mother Earth. Her approach is not that of a health food enthusiast, but rather that of a "natural goodness" enthusiast. At her cooking demonstrations she occasionally deplores the holier-than-thou attitude of health food proponents, pointing out that it is not necessary to shop in health food stores for the ingredients in her recipes. But *her main thrust is away from fabricated foods.*

More blows are being struck at cartoned carbohydrates everyday. But much more needs to be done in behalf of the birds, animals, and plants offered directly to you by Mother Earth.

Thousands of lobbyists for natural unprocessed foods are now being created by my books and by other high protein proponents.

They are good-looking slender people. They are the picture of good health. Their skin tone is radiant. They look youthful.

There will probably never be an organization that can have national publicity for the goodness of a soft-boiled egg, or a thick slab of rare roast beef, or of a salmon steak. So it is up to you.

As you now embark on the eating-est program of weight loss you ever dreamed possible, resolve to spread the word against manufactured foods and for natural proteins and produce.

Help balance the scales.

The Effect of Processed Carbohydrate Food on Weight

We use the term "processed food." What does that mean?

It generally means that it has been demineralized, devitaminized, and devitalized.

Processed largely means that anything alive in the food is taken out. That's so it won't "grow" on the shelves. It won't turn or spoil in any way. It won't attract worms or bugs or mould.

But the reason it now lasts on the shelves is that there's nothing left in it for the bugs to eat or for the mould to grow on.

It's dead food.

The processed foods line to the stomach

When your stomach gets it, the following conversation takes place:

> **Body**: Hey, stomach, send us all the nutrients you can out of that last shipment.
>
> **Stomach**: What nutrients? It's all carbohydrates. You'll have to use it for energy.
>
> **Body**: But we're still trying to get rid of the energy from this morning's carbohydrate shipment.
>
> **Stomach**: Sorry. I've churned it through several times. No nutrients. You'll just have to put it away in storage.
>
> **Body**: We're tight on storage space everywhere else, so keep it stored in your area.
>
> **Stomach**: Roger.

Suppose, in the above situation, energy was needed at the time? Would the body convert its fat? No, it would use this "shipment."

Suppose this was only a small meal and the body needed more energy than this supplied, would the body then convert its fat into energy?

It would depend . . .

If the body had not seen protein or nutrients for a long period, it would send out "fatigue" signs. The body would be saying, "Shortage of energy due to shortage of fat destroying supplies."

If the body had a liberal supply of protein and nutrients, yes, the body could then easily convert fat to energy.

FACT: Fat destroyer foods are also fat metabolizing foods.

Some Food Additives May Be Slow Killers

Besides devitalizing foods to make them keep longer, processors add chemicals.

Now, if these chemicals were just what the body needed, life would be rosy.

But these chemicals are just what the body does not need. And some of them are even suspected of causing serious diseases—and possible death.

Did you know that the simple process of homogenizing milk, so you don't have to shake it before pouring, destroys some of the valuable B vitamins and most of the C; and that the high pressures and temperatures used make the protein in milk less valuable to you by destroying an enzyme, called phosphatase, which is necessary for the body's absorption of phosphorus and calcium?

Some medical facts to consider

Speaking before the College of Medicine at the University of Iowa, Dr. Denis P. Burkitt revealed that cancer of the colon, unknown a century ago in the African villages from where American blacks were brought, began hitting one American black for every two whites 50 years ago, and today has achieved parity.

Dr. Burkitt, associated with the Medical Research Council of Great Britain, attributed this to the achievement of racial uniformity in the diet. He pointed to refined cereal in the American diet versus unrefined cereal, a staple in the African diet. With the unrefined cereal, he noted, roughage passed through the bowel faster, exposing it for shorter periods of time to carcinogenic agents. Some 20 percent of the adult population in the United States has polyps of the colon, but a research team in Johannesburg was able to find only six polyps after thirteen years of studying autopsy and biopsy material in a 2,500 bed hospital.

Processed Foods As a Cause of Obesity

Faulty nutrition—and I point the finger at foods with the good taken out and questionable chemicals substituted in their place—is a major cause of obesity. It is also a major cause of other serious illnesses.

I don't want to be morbid, but since I brought up cancer, let me remind you that extensive studies of the dietary habits of cancer patients suggest that people who are overweight past middle age are more likely to die of cancer than persons of normal weight or less. These findings are confirmed by surveys of life insurance statistics.

Sugar is a common additive used by food processors. It is cheap. It makes the food taste better. And it is a preservative. But, what else is sugar? Speaking before the National Health Federation, Victor H. Bagnall, D.O., said he believed sugar has caused more misery to the human race than any other one product.

He called sugar an irritant to the central nervous system. It stimulates the pancreas in a way that often produces hypo-glycemia and later diabetes. It also leaches out Vitamin B from body tissues.

Sugar is just one of scores of food additives that work against your natural good health and help to de-normalize your metabolism and your weight.

Are you aware of the controversy over cyclamates? Over monosodium glutamate? Over sodium nitrite? And these are only a few.

How about the long term effects of such questionable additives as the so-called U.S. certified food colorings and big sounding names like polysorbate, sorbitan-monosterate, sodium silico aluminate, carageenan and many others?

What's for dessert?

Here's a choice for your dessert.

a) A fresh grapefruit
b) A modern boxed dessert whip

Which do you take?
Even if they have the same number of carbo-cals, which they probably don't, your wise choice is the grapefruit.

A choice of dinner meat—read the labels on the package

Here is a choice for your dinner meat:

a) Broiled calf's liver
b) Baked ham from a can

Read the list of additives on the can. Do you need your proteins to be adulterated with these chemicals? The choice is fresh meat.
It's fine to read the labels on cans. But did you know that the Food and Drug Administration has four categories of ingredients: mandatory, permissible, unlabeled optional, and labeled optional. Applying this to cola drinks as an example, of 80 possible ingredients only one, caramel coloring, must appear on the label.
In many states, help for the consumer is on the way. There is a trend among large grocery chain producers toward open dating, comparative pricing, and nutritional labeling. The open dating removes the use of codes and permits the customer to see clearly when a product's freshness expires. The comparative pricing states the price per ounce for comparative shopping between sizes and brands. The nutritional labeling tells the customer the product's calories, vitamins, minerals, and other nutritional content.
Meanwhile . . . your choice should be as follows:
Choose fresh, unprocessed foods wherever you have that

choice—for a greater body ability to metabolize normally and move itself toward a normal weight.

High Protein Versus Low Carbohydrate

I have been describing the weight-loss program as a low carbohydrate diet.

From this page on, I want you to consider this instead as a high protein diet.

It isn't because I don't want to offend the carbohydrate interests. That die has long been cast.

I have a different purpose. It concerns you.

When you changed your way of eating in the past, it was always a case of sacrifice, of restriction, of giving up something.

You can sacrifice and restrict for only so long and then the effort ceases and the results are lost, the weight regained.

There is no such sacrifice facing you now.

However, to refer to a low "this diet," or a low "that diet" creates the impression that such a sacrifice is necessary.

No way. You eat like Henry VIII. So why give the diet a misleading name?

Fat destroying foods are great. The higher percentage of them you include in your daily input, the more fat they destroy.

Proteins are the key fat destroying foods. So this is a high protein fare.

Fat destroying foods that are not high in protein destroy fat because they are high in the minerals and nutrients needed by the body to carry on the complicated process of metabolizing fat away.

So your high protein diet is also a highly nutritional diet.

Why starve to lose weight when you can lose well while you eat well.

So, from here on, we avoid mentioning low carbohydrate in describing our fat destroying program. It's the high protein way.

The High Protein Diet That Is Almost "Free"

In the previous chapter, I gave you the Free Diet. It is a good one to start on as it involves the fewest changes, the least number of things to remember.

For most seriously overweight people, it is a good idea to start gradually and then shift into a higher gear, if the going gets slow.

The next higher gear is my standard High Protein Diet.

You may begin your weight loss program with this standard High Protein Diet, if you wish to save time and begin to burn off those pounds of fat at a good clip.

If you reach a plateau on this diet and wish to lose more, you can shift into the Higher Protein Diet, described in a later chapter, for stubborn pounds or faster weight loss, and finally a Highest Protein Diet for a few days of "crash" dieting.

Since the Free Diet was totally permissive except for two or three basic items, it took only a few sentences to spell out. The Standard High Protein Diet is quite free also, but requires more lists to describe it fully.

Here it is:

Standard High Protein Diet

You may eat: meat, fish, poultry, eggs, cheese prepared in any manner, but these may NOT be combined with carbohydrate products, i.e. flour, breading, sugar.

Salads, vegetables: You may choose any combination of these vegetables to make your salad (one average portion daily) and you may also choose your vegetables from this list (one average portion daily).

Asparagus	Eggplant	Radishes
Avocado	Endive	Sauerkraut
Bamboo Shoots	Escarole	Scallions
Bean Sprouts	Fennel	Spinach
Broccoli	Kale	String Beans
Brussels Sprouts	Lettuce	Summer Squash
Cabbage	Mushrooms	Tomatoes
Cauliflower	Okra	Turnips
Celery	Olives	Water Chestnuts
Chard	Onions	Water Cress
Chicory	Parsley	Wax Beans
Chinese Cabbage	Peppers) not sweet	Zucchini
Cucumber	Pickles)	

Fruits and fruit juices: One piece of fruit daily OR 6 ounces of any unsweetened fruit juice.

Beverages: Any liquid that is sugar free. *Milk:* Heavy or light cream—4 ounces daily. *Alcohol:* None.

Fats: You may use butter, margarine, oil, shortening, lard, mayonnaise.

Soups: Only if the ingredients contained in the soup are PERMITTED on this diet. (Read label carefully.)

Sauces, dressings, garnishes: You may use any combination of butter, eggs, egg yolks, cream, lemon or lime juice, parsley, any sugarless seasonings, grated fruit rind, sour cream, horseradish, scallions, garlic, chives, vinegar, grated onion, beef or chicken seasonings, Tabasco sauce, Worcestershire sauce, soy sauce, mustard, dill, mayonnaise, crumbled bacon or pork rind, grated cheese, mushrooms, anchovies, minced ham, chicken, turkey, cheese, tongue, roast beef.

You Can Lose Weight on Second and Third Portions, Five and Six Meals a Day

As you can see, more restrictions go into effect on the standard High Protein Diet compared to the Free Diet:

- One average portion of salad daily.
- One average portion of vegetable daily.
- One piece of fruit daily, or 6 ounces of unsweetened fruit juice.
- No alcohol.
- No milk, but up to 4 ounces of heavy or light cream.

However, again I ask you accent the positive—to look at what you can eat, instead of what you can't:

- There are no restrictions on the number of meals you can have each day.
- There are no restrictions on the number of portions of meat, fish, poultry, eggs, or cheese you can enjoy in those meals.

Does this look like a diet?

Breakfast—6-ounce glass of fresh orange juice, 3 fried eggs, 4 slices of bacon, coffee with heavy cream.

Second Breakfast—3 link sausages, coffee with heavy cream.

Lunch—Hamburger steak (¼ pound, ½ pound, ¾ pound—you name it), mixed salad greens with mayonnaise dressing. Coffee with heavy cream.

Second Lunch—Leftover hamburger steak, coffee with heavy cream.

Dinner—Roast leg of lamb (two portions), brussels sprouts, selected cheeses, coffee with heavy cream.

Late Snack—Cold lamb.

You Can Almost See Your Body Jettison Its Fat

It is most certainly a diet. Overweight people lose on this diet every day.

If you were to add up the calories, you would find over 2,000 and possibly over 2,500. But this total is not the key.

The key to its weight-losing effectiveness is the fact that there are less than 200 carbo-cals.

Contributing to these carbo-cals are the juice, the vegetable, and the salad, in that order.

All of the other foods are fat destroying foods when deprived of the presence of these carbo-cals.

Check your urine with that little stick, if you don't believe that the high protein count is causing your body to jettison its fat.

Ninety percent of the standard High Protein Diet consists of fat destroying foods.

Ninety-five percent of the Higher Protein Diet is fat destroying foods.

One hundred percent of the Highest Protein (Crash) Diet is fat destroying foods.

The greater the percent of fat destroying foods, the more effective your menus are in causing your scale to move in the direction you want.

Quantity of food counts. Quantity, however, is not the critical factor as it is in the conventional carbohydrate-heavy diets, now fast becoming obsolete.

Quantity becomes more critical as weight approaches normalcy.

Fat Destroying Foods Act as Appetite Depressants

As we mentioned before, carbohydrates give you quick energy. They move through the digestive system rapidly and provide blood sugar, often within a few minutes, certainly within an hour or two.

But then you are hungry again.

The expression that protein foods "stick to your ribs" is ill-chosen. Carbohydrate foods stick to your ribs—and your buttocks, hips, and points south.

Protein foods do remain in your stomach longer. They take longer to be digested.

You do not feel hungry when your stomach is still busy at work.

Few people on the standard High Protein Diet will feel the need to eat as much as shown on the sample menus listed on pp. 133-146.

Coffee breaks, second breakfasts and late snacks have been spawned largely from our modern doughnuts and Danish society.

Our grandparents, who enjoyed sometimes as many as a half dozen meats for breakfast, never came back for a second breakfast. Their high protein days permitted them to work hard for longer hours without the need for "breaks" or "snacks."

So a happy by-product of the High Protein Diet is a lessened need for quantity and frequency.

You can eat all you want.

But you want less.

You can eat as frequently as hunger strikes.

But hunger strikes less frequently.

Conflicting rules for long, healthy life

People are built differently. Their metabolisms are different. Their needs are different. Not everyone can succeed on the High Protein Diet. They may not get results until they move to the Higher Protein Diet. Or their systems may not be able to handle these types of diets at all. That is why I keep advising you to stay under your physician's observation as you proceed.

A survey, over the years, of people over one hundred years of age has turned up the following differences in their secrets for long life.

Get plenty of sleep—10 or 12 hours per day.
Sleep only four hours a day.

Don't eat meat.
Eat a pound of meat a day.

Abstain from alcohol.
Drink a pint of brandy or whiskey a day

Avoid sexual activity.
Be sexually active.

Don't eat dairy products.
Eat only butter, eggs, cheese, and milk.

Don't satisfy all your appetites; use self-discipline
Eat all you want, whenever you want it.

They say one man's meat is another man's poison. They should also say one man's potato is another man's poison.

You are a special person. You have to see what works for you. You don't have to be a hundred years old to find out. You'll know now.

Under your physician's watchful eye, you can try the Free Diet, then the standard High Protein Diet. If you feel fine, and the scale shows results, stay with it. Additional menus for the High Protein Diet are in a subsequent chapter.

Children and the High Protein Diet

Children are special people, too. Unfortunately, the carbohydrate food interests look upon children as special customers. "Hook 'em on sugar while they are young. Hey, Mom, give the kid some cookies so you can have some time to yourself." So it has gone, but let's hope it does not go thus in your home.

Statistics show that plump children grow into overweight people more often than not. Most fat cells, once created, stay with us. When the fat disappears visibly, it's because the fat cells shrink, not because they are eliminated.

So when fat is destroyed, the fat "receptacle" merely empties and waits to be refilled.

That's one reason for the yo-yo syndrome. Once you have been overweight, it is easier to gain ten pounds than if you are starting from what has been a permanently slender shape.

Why it's important to get children to remain at their correct weight

It is, therefore, especially important for children to remain at their proper weight. A few pounds of extra fat cells now can spell years of weight problems for them in the future.

Start with your infant.

Sure, those little jars of baby food on the supermarket shelf are tempting. Just twist off the lid, heat it if you're in the mood, and spoon it into baby's mouth—the emulsifiers, the preservatives, the monosodium glutamate, the sugar, the colorants, the modified starch.

Down it goes. That's a good child. What do you care; it's easy. And don't millions of babies "thrive" on it?

So the ads say. But do they? Ask your pediatrician.

Recently, in a span of eight months, three books[1] were published on this subject, two by individuals and one by a husband-wife team, all concerned with the feeding of their own children.

The books all agree that it is safer and more nutritionally beneficial—as well as more economical—to prepare your own infant foods.

This preparation need not be a separate operation. Some of the family roast and vegetables can be separated before being fancied up with spices, then placed in a blender for baby.

Of the three books, the Turners' book is the most critical of the baby food industry. Mr. Turner, a Washington attorney, was project director for a Ralph Nader report entitled "The Chemical

---

[1] *The First Babyfood Cookbook,* Melinda Morris, New York: Grosset and Dunlap. *Feeding Your Baby the Safe and Healthy Way,* Ruth Pearlman, New York: Random House. *Making Your Own Baby Food,* John and Mary Turner, New York: Workman Publishing Company.

Feast." He hits hard at the industry's trying to justify their use of additives.

So much for baby food. When the infant is old enough to watch television, he is then subjected to the carbohydrate bombardment directly. He begins to get his basic nutritional education and it all points to:

> Eat cereal, cookies, candy, and sweet drinks all day. If you are not hungry for your regular meal, don't worry, you can have a cracker or two later.

It has been reported that on a Saturday morning in New York, of 388 network commercials during 29 hours of children's programs, 82 percent were for candy, gum, food, drink, and vitamin pills.

If you were to monitor your own Saturday morning programs with the help of your neighbors, you would find uncle and daddy-type salesmen sweet talking your kids into sugared breakfast cereals, frozen waffles, pop tarts, canned pasta, frozen dinners, canned desserts, sodas and beverage mixes, popcorn, candy, and other snacks.

Little wonder that when regular meal time arrives eggs don't fit in the picture, cheese is a no-no, and chicken seems unappetizing.

I resolve that when television sets are modified to accept your own video tapes, I'm going to make such a tape. I'll dress in a clown suit and sell your kids calf's liver and turnip greens.

Hone Up Your Own Knowledge of Proteins

Children need to be made aware of the value of proteins. You are the only source of this information for them, until they get beyond the primary grades.

But you, the teacher, need to keep at least a lesson or two ahead of your pupils. Here are some of the main points to get across to yourself first.

- Proteins are made up of complex nutrients called amino acids. Like building blocks, they create and re-create your body.
- Plants can manufacture proteins but they are not complete proteins. When you eat an incomplete plant protein (as in soy beans), it will

repair worn out tissue in the body, but it won't create new tissue. So a child cannot grow on plant protein alone.

- Animals that eat incomplete plant protein convert it to complete protein. Animals cannot make protein in their bodies from what they eat, but they can "finish" proteins "started" by plants.
- Man cannot make protein either. But he can use incomplete plant protein for repair. For growth, he needs to get complete proteins. For these, he must depend largely on animals. So he needs to drink milk and eat dairy products from cows, eat eggs from chickens, and enjoy steak, liver, and other meats from farm animals and chickens. These are complete proteins necessary to grow new tissue. One exception is the glutenin of wheat. It contains all essential amino acids, but it is part of a largely carbohydrate food.
- You don't need carbohydrates for energy. Proteins do just as well. Each grain of carbohydrate produces four calories of energy. So does each grain of protein. Proteins do not turn to fat as readily as carbohydrates if there is an excess. Nor is it as easily stored by the body. Only 60 percent of protein excess can become fat, whereas 100 percent of unused carbohydrates can become fat—and usually does.

The digestion and metabolism of protein, fat, and carbohydrate is a complicated subject. "It is believed" appears as frequently as "it has been shown," if you read the texts.

Perhaps, it's just as well. We are justified then in approaching the subject from an experiential rather than intellectual basis:

Enjoy a high protein diet. See what it does for your digestion. See what it does for your energy level. See what it does for your disposition.

And see what it does for your weight.

Lose 1 Percent of Your Weight Per Week

Half of the overweight people who go on the standard High Protein Diet find that it takes them all the way to their normal weight.

The rest find that they reach a plateau where weight loss ceases (and may even rise somewhat).

If you reach a point where you do not register a weight loss for one week, prepare to shift diets. The safe loss of weight is 1 percent of your weight per week. More than this means you should consider restoring some carbohydrates. Less than this means you better sharpen your carbohydrate cutter.

Your next stop is the Higher Protein Diet. Still loads of delicious dishes to highlight your breakfasts, lunches, and dinners. Still no hunger, no deprivation.

But you are getting into a highly disciplined area,—one where the guard is doubled to keep out every possible carbohydrate intruder.

And you are getting into a temporary mode of eating,—a diet in the true sense of the word. In other words, you will be ending the Higher Protein Diet at some time, whereas you can stay on the High Protein Diet forever.

All is not lost, though. You are not going to be faced with regaining any lost weight. The reason is the High Protein Diet will back you up.

When you return to the High Protein Diet, you will stop losing, but you will be able to maintain your normal weight. It is a maintenance diet and so it is not a diet in the discredited sense.

It is, rather, a way of life.

And what a life! New vigor, new youth, new self-confidence, new friends, new attraction.

New horizons, basically for your full measure of satisfaction and happiness.

5

THE HIGHER PROTEIN AND
HIGHEST PROTEIN (CRASH) DIETS

So far—no hunger pangs for you in this book's eating program. Plenty of steaming hot food, delicious cold snacks.

And fat anchors away.

In this chapter, you can lose faster but, for some, there may be hunger at times.

No hunger for most while on the Higher Protein Diet, as it differs only very slightly from the High Protein Diet. The difference is one hundred carbo-cals less (which you can make up for with two hundred prote-cals more, if you wish). And we bear down just a bit on the fats.

On the other hand, for the Highest Protein (Crash) Diet, hunger is the name of the game.

However, this Crash Diet is for stubborn cases and is not meant to be used for more than a few days, or possibly a week, and then only under your physician's supervision.

"I Don't Know Why I Eat—It's Not Because I'm Hungry"

Proteins not only destroy fat, they shatter hunger. They stay in your stomach twice as long as carbohydrates to prevent that empty, gnawing feeling.

But many people don't need that empty, gnawing feeling to feel "hungry." They eat, not because their stomach is empty, but because their spirits are low.

"I'm Not Hungry, but I Look for Something to Eat"

Betty is married to a man who travels. Although this has been the case for many years, Betty has simply never been able to get used to it. When her husband is out of town, she is lonely and depressed. When she is lonely and depressed, she eats and eats and eats.

In her own words, "I am always all right in the daytime but once the evening starts, I begin my walk back and forth to the refrigerator. Sometimes I will finish a whole cake. I am not hungry but I am always looking for something to eat. Last night, knowing I was coming to see you today, I ate a whole quart of chocolate ice cream. I do not eat because I am hungry. I don't know why I eat."

Betty's case is typical of thousands who repeat the same words, "I don't eat because I am hungry." There are many reasons that people eat when they are not hungry. For example, if you are in a restaurant and have finished your appetizer, soup, and main course, you certainly are not hungry. Yet, when the waiter hands you a dessert menu or, even worse, when he rolls the dessert wagon to your table and you choose that succulent sweet to finish your meal, you are eating without being hungry.

Foods are enjoyable not only to satisfy hunger but for their taste value and their differences in hot or cold, sweet or sour, soft or crisp. Taste changes and textures make foods attractive, largely because they satisfy sensory or emotional needs. Only once in a while do we eat because we are truly hungry. Most other times we eat because it is time to eat or because something we thought of, saw, or smelled tickled our appetite palate.

Betty is, in reality, a victim of conditioning. She, like millions of others, conditioned herself to replace one emotion with another. In this particular case, loneliness with self-gratification. The mood that she experienced while eating temporarily gratified her emotional emptiness.

Unfortunately, it also made her fat.

Betty came to see me because she realized it was time for her to make some changes. First, she had to realize the necessity of recognizing the situation as it really was. Her husband was not choosing to be out of town in preference to being with her. She also had to realize that she was fooling herself thinking that dieting minimally during the day, but stuffing herself at night, would produce a weight loss. Also, it was not really the amount of food she was eating at night but the type of food.

By adjusting her diet to breakfast, lunch and dinner menus high in protein and allowing late night snacks (as indicated in Chapter 7 menus), Betty was able to enjoy her meals and her snacks and lose weight. Most important was Betty's recognition of the way her emotions were leading her to the refrigerator.

Diet Pills Create More Problems Than Solutions

A cartoon recently caused a national smile when it depicted a very stout man receiving a bottle of pills from his doctor. They are not for eating, explains the doctor, just spill them on the floor once a day and pick them up one at a time.

That's about the best dietary use for amphetamines and other pills that I've come across.

The late magazine *Life* ran a feature on the multihued diet pills that many doctors dispense. Some, it pointed out, have no effect. Others can be dangerous combinations of amphetamines, thyroid extract, and other materials. There are combinations of these pills that could be deadly.

More often than not, these pills rely on the "upper" or "downer" effect. The "uppers" give you a synthetic lift and relieve you of depressed feelings that you might otherwise seek to relieve in the kitchen. The "downers" depress the metabolism and the appetite.

Pills are not the "easy way"

Some so-called obesity specialists dispense pills and capsules in their reducing "factories" often with only superficial examination. Patients walk out with phenobarbital, amphetamines, laxatives, dehydrating agents, and appetite depressants, thinking they have the easy way finally to lose weight.

The results are serious enough to trigger periodic investigations by Congress and other government agencies. I know one such dispenser of pills who is hooked on his own drugs.

I say dispense *with* them.

You will not be hungry on the Higher Protein Diet. Again, you can eat all you want of eggs and breakfast meats in the morning; fish, cheeses, poultry, or meat for lunch; steaks, roasts, and gourmet-high protein dishes at dinner.

But "all you want" now needs to be more closely aligned to physical needs rather than mental illusions of physical needs.

Before you go on the Higher Protein Diet, give some thought to why you eat as much as you do. Such self-examination can have a much more immediate effect than any appetite-depressant or other diet pill yet invented.

What Happens to Your Extra Pounds When You Increase Protein Percentage

The Higher Protein Diet does not mean that you must eat more proteins. It means that you must eat less carbohydrates and preferably also less fat.

This decrease of fat and carbohydrates increases the percentage that protein constitutes of your total intake.

This percentage is the weight regulator. The less carbohydrate, the faster the weight loss. The resulting higher protein percentage, the greater the destruction of unwanted fat.

Of course, quantity reduction helps, too. In Chapter 11, I repeat all three high protein diets with a restrictive point system whereby you can accelerate weight loss two ways—by cutting down points and by cutting down carbohydrates as we are now doing.

In his book "Physiology of Man,"[1] L.L. Langley, Ph.D., states that every reducing diet should have an unusually high protein content. He points up both the need of protein for maintenance of

[1] Van Nostrand Reinhold Company, New York, N.Y.

vital tissues and the special way that proteins keep the metabolic rate elevated.

We are now going to get into unusually high protein diets indeed.

The Higher Protein Diet is about 95% protein and fat. The Highest Protein (Crash) Diet is as close to 100% protein and fat as you can get.

Again I say, consult with your physician before embarking on even these temporary programs. They are not for everyone.

Natives of areas where fish and game provide the sole subsistence live in excellent health on a near 100 percent protein fare. Eskimos, who live on high fat diets, are healthy people. The only people who develop degenerative diseases and fill hospitals to overflowing are civilized people who subsist on highly refined carbohydrate diets.

On a diet of 95 percent protein and fat, you will lose weight faster than on the High Protein Diet which was 85 to 90 percent protein and fat. The estimated increased loss: one pound a week. This means a loss of up to three pounds a week for a woman and up to four pounds a week for a man, depending, too, on total weight.

Two Rules to Remember

Rule 1. When you want to increase protein percentage, you should cut down on carbohydrates first, fats next.
Rule 2. When you want to accelerate weight loss, you should increase protein percentage first, decrease total intake next.

Rule 1 is implemented by the High, Higher, and Highest (Crash) Protein Diets described in Chapters 4 and 5.

Rule 2 is implemented by the precision Point System outlined in Chapter 11.

When you increase protein percentage to the limit, you are eating a maximum of fat destroying foods and a minimum of fat creating foods.

From then on, there is no place to go except to reduce total intake. You may never have to reach Chapter 11 where total intake is reduced. There is likelihood that you will reach your normal weight on the Higher Protein Diet (eat all you want) with a possible temporary assist from the Highest (Crash) Protein Diet.

The Higher Protein Diet

The Higher Protein Diet contains very few changes from the High Protein Diet in Chapter 4.

These changes reduce carbo-cals from a maximum of 200 to a maximum of 100. They also seek to reduce fat calories. These are all replaced by fat destroying prote-cals.

There is no limit on protein foods in the Higher Protein Diet. Here is the daily diet in a nutshell:

You may eat unrestrictedly of:

Fish	Eggs
Poultry	Meat
Cheese	

You may drink unrestrictedly of:

Water	Diet sodas
Coffee	Other sugar-free beverages
Tea	(No fruit juices or alcoholic beverages)

You may eat cautiously:

Vegetables	(one modest portion from the list that follows)
Fruit	(one medium piece of fruit or melon or medium portion of berries)
Salad	(one portion from the list that follows)
Fats and oils	(salad oil and mayonnaise are permitted, but curb heavy cream)

Salads—Vegetables

Asparagus	Cucumber	Radishes
Bamboo Shoots	Eggplant	Sauerkraut
Bean Sprouts	Endive	Scallions

Salads—Vegetables *(cont.)*

Beet Greens	Escarole	Soy Beans
Broccoli	Fennel	Spinach
Brussels Sprouts	Kale	String Beans
Cabbage	Lettuce (all types)	Summer Squash
Cauliflower	Mushrooms	Tomatoes
Celery	Okra	Turnips
Chard	Onions	Turnip Greens
Chicory	Parsley	Water Chestnuts
Chinese Cabbage	Peppers) not sweet	Watercress
Chives	Pickles)	Zucchini

The menus in Chapter 7 can help you glamorize fat destroyer foods and vary your daily meals and snacks. You will note that the righthand column provides you with Higher Protein Diet ideas, by merely making a few substitutions in the basic High Protein Diet.

You can still enjoy sizzling platters of bacon and eggs in the morning. Large hamburger steaks or tuna fish salads for lunch. Roasts and barbeques for dinner. Cold meats and cheeses in between meals.

Special Advice

If you want the Higher Protein Diet to take you the rest of the way to your normal weight, so that you don't have to go on the more restrictive Crash Diet or Precision Point System, then here is my advice to you:

- Select your fat destroyer foods from the higher protein items under meat, poultry, fish, and cheeses.
- Watch vegetables and fruit portions extremely carefully. (Remember, no fruit juices, just whole fruit.)
- Go easy on the salad dressing.
- Favor meat over cheese and eggs.
- Enjoy your coffee black for awhile.
- Stay off alcoholic beverages for this period.
- Take vitamins and mineral supplements.
- Remain under your physician's supervision.

Losing Weight Too Fast

There is such a thing as losing weight too fast. One percent of your weight per week is a good, safe rule of thumb to follow. Two percent a week should be considered the top limit, one at which you should not remain too long.

If you are losing weight too fast, shift back to the High Protein Diet.

If you are still not losing weight fast enough. . . .

Shift to the Highest Protein Diet for a Crash Program

Arthur was an attorney. He was 31-years old, 5'9" tall, and weighed 297 pounds. During the past ten years, his lowest weight had been between 215 and 220 pounds. He wanted to get down to 190 pounds. I allowed that was a good start.

Arthur blamed his excessive weight on his irregular working hours and the pace involved. He told me that there were days when he lived on a few candy bars and perhaps some nuts for good measure. When he finally got home at night, he just did not seem to be able to stop eating. His dinner always included a rich dessert—pie, ice cream, and the like. His motivation to diet was lessened by a resigned feeling because his family had a history of obesity.

In order to shock him into a limited food intake, I put him on the Highest Protein (Crash) Diet. If he could not leave his office, he was instructed to send someone out to get him foods that were on his list.

I was somewhat pessimistic about his case because it did not mean merely a change in dietary habits but actually in a way of life. To my great satisfaction, however, Arthur seemed to take his dieting quite seriously. He lost 15 pounds the first week.

I thought it best then to shift him to the Higher Protein Diet. His weight continued the downward trend at the rate of 10 to 12 pounds a month, so that in about a year he had reached his goal.

Here is the Highest Protein Diet. It is a crash program. Go on it only with medical supervision. Stay on it a week at the most:

You may eat restrictedly *three times a day* of:

Beef (lean cuts only, 4 ounces)
Cheese (3 ounces)
Poultry (6 ounces)
Fish (6 ounces)
Cottage Cheese (6 ounces)

Coffee, tea, water, calorie-free sodas are unlimited.
No other foods are allowed.
I repeat: this diet is not recommended for extended use.
Well, we got into the old starvation trip after all. But let's hope that it's only for a few days if you ever have to go to this extreme at all.

Cases for a Crash Diet Program

My clients seldom need this crash program. Those who do fall into the following categories:

- Those who need to lose a few stubborn pounds to reach their normal weight.
- Models, actresses, jockeys, etc. who have to meet certain low weight requirements.
- Overweight people who need a dietary "shock" to change their bad eating habits.
- Those on other high protein diets who reach a plateau or who are losing too slowly.

How a Stewardess Lost Weight and Regained Her Job

Mary was employed as a stewardess on an airline and was currently on probation. Her sin: overweight. She was frustrated and angry.

Since her marriage two years before, Mary had started to blossom out. She had watched herself much more carefully before she was married but now things were out of hand. She had been warned by her employer and she had tried, but to no avail.

She was one of the women I see quite frequently who could literally add a pound to her weight by eating a slice of chocolate cake. Statistically, this is quite impossible, as an average wedge of chocolate cake contains approximately 350 calories. Theoretically, it could add 1.6 ounces of weight. But, in Mary's case, as in the case of other people I dub the "fatten easilys," it could literally add ten times that,—a full pound. I can't explain the metabolic process. Let's just call it "fatabolism." Mary was one of those carbohydrate "allergic" people and was unable to lose weight even on a balanced 1,200 calorie diet.

It was necessary to lose weight quickly and she started immediately on the Highest Protein (Crash) Diet. Three days later, she phoned me tearfully. "I have not lost an ounce!" I explained to her that this was not unusual. I assured her that the under-pinnings of her avoirdupois were being loosened. "Hang on a few days," I urged her, "The pounds will soon be tumbling off."

She was due in my office four days later and when she came through the door, I could see immediately that success was at hand. She had lost her bloated look. She cheerfully announced that the morning after her telephone call, which was on the fourth day of her diet, she had lost five pounds. She had, in fact, lost more weight in the eight days on my Highest Protein (Crash) Diet than she had lost in a month on a 1,200 calorie "balanced" diet.

Mary is back now to the protein maintenance diet, which is the same as the Free Diet in Chapter 4, and she is happily pouring the coffee at 35,000 feet.

Crash Program Tricks That Beat Hunger

Every Christmas, clergymen around the country receive gifts from their parishioners. Although meant in kindness, these gifts are Trojan horses. One Texas physician reported that his pastor received over thirty pounds of chocolates, countless fruit cakes, a score or more of "tons" of homemade chocolate fudge, and dozens of pies, layer cakes, and jars of honey, jellies and jams, not to speak of the flood of cookies. Rather than have their pastor robbed of his health, the physician convinced the community the following year to contribute toward a summer vacation for the pastor and his family.

The question comes to mind: was the pastor really free of such goodies the next Christmas or had a habit set in? The goodies could have still been his holiday hallmark either by dint of his own habit pattern or that of many of his parishioners.

Habits play tricks on our resolve and on our appetite.

But we can play tricks, too, and beat the simulated hunger that habit creates.

Habits are created by repeated behavior. The repetition sets up circuits in our brain that are triggered by a stimulus.

For instance, if we are in the habit of retiring at 10:00 p.m., when that time arrives we feel sleepy. It does not matter whether we have had an easy day or a hard day. The stimulus that triggers the yawn is the arrival of 10:00 p.m.

If we are in the habit of eating at certain times during the day, we feel hungry at those times. It does not matter whether we have had a snack a couple of hours ago or not. The stimulus has occurred and the circuit is activated.

If we are on the crash diet calling for three meals a day, but we are "wired" for morning coffees and afternoon teas, we are going to be "bugged" to eat at those extra times, too. The trick is to eat at all the times you are "wired" to eat at, even if it means splitting a six-ounce portion of fish or cottage cheese.

The Precision Point System

The Precision Point System explained in Chapter 11 provides an example of how the Crash Diet can be divided over six meals a day.

The place we eat is another "mental circuit." If we pass a luncheonette where we frequently pop in for a snack, we are going to be motivated to eat every time we pass it. The trick is to take a different route.

Stay out of your kitchen as much as you can for those few days you are on the Crash Diet. Let someone else do the cooking, or at least the cleaning up.

We are also wired to require certain size portions. If the mouth doesn't chomp up and down the usual number of times, the stomach sends out a hunger signal.

So fool it. Eat more slowly and retain each mouthful longer, chewing better and savoring more.

How to Rewire Your Appetite Circuits

Suppose you were sitting watching the late evening news on television and decided that it was time to go to bed. Suppose, too, that you remember the leftover pie you had for dinner. It's in an aluminum pie dish, covered by a plastic wrap and nearly half of it is left. How about a slice? No, you say,—had two pieces for dinner. Does it end there? Not on your life. Rare is the willpower that can beat a visual image.

Once you visualize something, you are triggering one of those behavior circuits in the brain.

A Practical Example of Visualization Control

Try this one. Visualize what you now read:

Some friends are visiting you and have brought some "goodies." On the dining table is a chocolate cake. It looks beautiful. As you approach it you see to your consternation that it is crawling with cockroaches. The cake is actually alive with bugs!

Now, if you have visualized that picture realistically and if somebody walked through the door right now and offered you a piece of chocolate cake, would you be tempted? Chances are you would not only feel no temptation, you would find the cake repugnant to you.

People are your worst diet breakers. They say, "Come on, one slice won't hurt." And, as in the case of the pastor, they bring you "goodies."

If you can't say no to your friends or family, play a mental trick on them. You don't have to visualize cockroaches, but if somebody pushes food at you that you don't need, see it in some unappetizing way. Maybe it is mouldy, tainted, or rancid. One effective image is to see it as turning to fat the minute it trickles down your throat.

You can do this visualizing in these preventive ways but you can also utilize them in reinforcing ways.

If you want the Crash Diet to be easier for you, sit right down where you are, read these instructions, put the book down, and then visualize accordingly.

This works best if you are in a thoroughly relaxed position, so make sure you are comfortably seated in the chair. Loosen any tight clothing. Take your shoes off if that will make you feel better.

Take a deep breath to relax you further,—like the deep sigh of relief that you sometimes exhale.

Now see yourself going through a day on the Crash Program. See yourself thoroughly satisfied after a two-egg breakfast, going through to lunch with no hunger, enjoying a cottage cheese lunch, and then a hamburger steak dinner with no desire for "in-betweens." See yourself getting on the scale each day. See the scale registering less weight each time. See yourself looking more slender. See yourself happier and healthier.

Ready? Put the book down, relax, and visualize. . . .

Mental Food That Can Be More Nourishing Than Stomach Food

Brandi was 100 percent proof that the mind can make us over-weight and the mind can make us slim. Born Beatrice, a name which she hated, she renamed herself Brandi on her college application forms. The name Beatrice was just one of her hatreds. She also hated the government, the police department, her relatives, and the male chauvinist dictates that had cunningly infiltrated into her world.

At age 28, she had a pretty face but a not so pretty body. She was probably 75 pounds overweight. I say probably because she refused to get on the scale in front of me. She would weigh herself only if I left her alone in the small room where the scale was located. She would always sweep the weight bars back to zero before she left the room.

Brandi's mental state—and her fatness

At college, she had been an "A" student and had made the Dean's List each year. She had always been heavy, even as a child, never really knowing what it was like to be of normal weight. She had grown up during the "do your own thing" era and had gone through the drug scene, the free-love scene, and "all adults are hypocrites" scene.

Her current gripe was that she was not getting any acceptance. She was being turned down by prospective employers, men, and contemporaries. She displayed her resentment against all these rejections by eating up a storm.

The more she ate, the fatter she got. The fatter she got, the more she felt rejected. And the more she felt rejected, the more she ate.

It never seemed to strike her that she was being rejected largely because of her weight. Instead, she developed an obnoxious and hostile personality.

I had long talks with Brandi. We talked about the fallacies in the "Establishment." In today's competitive world there is no shortage of good typists or executives, no shortage of receptionists or management positions. Appearance is, and always has been, an asset and it often is a decisive factor. Whether that be right or wrong, it is so. Until it changes, it is going to be extremely frustrating to buck the system.

Overweight also creates changes in personality. It is a contributing cause of protective defense systems, of sensitivity, and of hostility. We know we are not the image of youthfulness, vitality, health, and slenderness that the whole world admires.

Brandi wanted to be accepted as an intelligent, industrious woman. But she did not see what her weight had to do with her capabilities. She was right, but the cost of being right was proving too expensive in happiness.

It took a great deal of effort for Brandi to recognize that, right or wrong, her weight was a major deterrent to her happiness. But once she got turned on, she was as impatient to lose the weight as she was impatient with most things in her life. Her new insight helped her to go on and stay on the Crash Diet. It did wonders for her. So did her new outlook.

The emotional key

At Honolulu's Straub Clinic, a group of stubbornly overweight patients, mostly in the 200 to 250 pounds category, discovered that by examining their emotions instead of their stomach they could lose weight.

This inside-out approach was successful for all but one who dropped out. The program, conducted under the supervision of Dr. Edwin Gramlich, the Clinic's chief of psychiatry, has discovered that people overeat because they are missing some kind of satisfaction. With some it's the satisfaction of being financially secure, with others the missing satisfaction could be sex, affection, tenderness.

Once this missing satisfaction is identified and supplied, the need to supply it with food is ended. This is not always easy. If it is a marital situation, it takes cooperation by two people to solve the problem.

Also, an overweight person is often unaware that there is any problem to begin with. Are you frustrated? No, I'm hungry. Are you lonely? No, I'm hungry. Are you angry? No, I'm hungry.

Many do not differentiate between hunger and their emotions. The frustration, loneliness, anger actually ring the hunger bell. Perhaps, it's a way of shifting the pain from some insoluble problem to one that is easily soluble in the digestive juices.

Emotions masquerading as hunger

The advantage of the Straub Clinic project is that its patients relearn to identify the feeling masquerading as hunger. They learn to express frustration, express loneliness, and express anger. This is done through group sessions wherein the patients relate to each other and through this inter-action—this ability to talk about their personal feelings—they begin to express those feelings less inhibitedly.

Diet pills are not used. The Clinic long recognized the ineffectiveness of diet pills, even before a government-appointed panel of consultants concluded most were clinically trivial, and that their slight short-term weight effects were negligible compared to the high potential for abuse and physical damage.

I recommend this "head first" approach. If you can understand why you overeat, you have a better chance of combating the carbohydrate attack on you, of studying with fat destroyer foods, and of sticking to the Crash Diet if you have to.

You do not need a group to discover your inner secrets. You can identify missing satisfactions yourself by pausing to study the circumstances at the moment of your urge to overeat or eat wrong foods.

Or, you can form a group of your friends who are interested in successful, permanent weight loss. There are books available that provide interesting psychological games you can play in such sessions to make you more aware of each other and of yourself.[2]

Start with the Free Diet
Not with the Crash Diet

Well, there you are.

I cannot cut carbo-cals any further or I'd have another high protein diet for you.

The only next step is the Precision Point System in Chapter 11, which places quantity intake under more strict controls—easy controls that give you a way to adjust your weight loss—slow it or accelerate it, merely by adding or subtracting points.

I have placed the Free Diet first in this book (Chapter 3) because you should try this approach before going on to more stringent methods.

If weight loss is not satisfactory in a few days, shift to the High Protein Diet (Chapter 4). You may be able to reach your goal on this diet. If not, then go on to the Higher Protein Diet in this chapter, and, as a last resort to get that fat destroyed—the Crash Diet.

In some of the cases I related to you, I mentioned that I put the person on the Crash Diet right off the bat. These were special cases and a matter of considered judgement on my part at the time. Save the Crash Diet as a last resort for you.

---

[2]"Conduct Your Own Awareness Sessions,"Christopher B. Hills and Robert B. Stone, New American Library, N.Y.

In the next chapter are the protein, fat, and carbohydrate food tables, with menus in Chapter 7 and gourmet recipes in Chapter 8—all featuring fat destroying foods.

Take a look in the mirror today.

You'll begin to acquire a new look tomorrow.

6

COMPLETE TABLE OF PROTEIN,
FAT AND CARBOHYDRATE CONTENT
OF COMMON FOODS

"Cottage cheese is very high in protein."

"No, it isn't. It contains lots of carbo-cals."

Two women were looking over a luncheon menu when this question arose. They were both experienced dieters, having been on and off the best of them. Yet, they disagreed about the dietary nature of as common a diet food as cottage cheese.

The fact is that the usual uncreamed variety of cottage cheese is low in fat and therefore low in total calories. That is what makes it a popular diet item.

As to its protein-carbohydrate content, of the 195 calories in a one cup portion, 24 of these are carbo-cals. This isn't bad, but it's bad enough to throw your carbo-cal limit off if you don't know about it. Most cheeses are much lower in carbo-cals per portion.

To help you select the right foods for your fat destroying menus, I have, in the pages ahead, provided you with the protein, fat, and carbohydrate content of some five hundred common foods.

Now these tables can be very valuable to you if you know how to use them. They have been adapted from values supplied by the United States Department of Agriculture.

Let's look at each of the seven columns to see how we can benefit from the table. Starting from the left:

Column One. These are the particular food items. They are grouped in categories, such as VEGETABLES AND VEGETABLE PRODUCTS or MILK, CREAM, CHEESE, RELATED PRODUCTS. Under some of these categories, there are sub-categories. If you are looking up a special food, such as cottage cheese, you will find it in its proper category and sub-category but do not expect to find it in alphabetical order. That is because the foods have been arranged in protein order instead (see explanation for column three).

Column Two. This spells out the quantity. I have not used grams or some other impractical measurement but have tried to stick to cup, ounce, slice, etc. to make your average portion more easily gauged. Note that cottage cheese appears as one cup, whereas other cheeses are measured by the ounce.

Column Three. This is the total calories or food energy content. This is where most calorie tables stop. Cottage cheese, one cup—195 calories. But what kind of calories are they?

Column Four. This is perhaps the most informative column of all for the person on a high protein program. It reveals the protein percentage. To the right, in column five, are the protein calories. Column four is the percentage there is of the total calories shown in column three. Since high protein is critical, the foods in each sub-category are placed in order of the highest percentage of protein, with the lowest protein percentage last. However, there is need to examine column seven, too, in selecting foods, as low carbohydrate content is even more important than high protein content. Like cottage cheese, a 78 percent protein food may have most of the other 22 percent in carbohydrates. Or, like roast beef, the rest could be in fat with no carbo-cals at all.

Column Five. If you multiply the total calories in column three by the protein percentage in column four, you get the protein calories in column five. These are fat destroying calories.

Column Six. These are the number of fat calories in the portion shown.

Column Seven. These are the villains of our story. Here are the carbo-cals that are the hooks for unwanted pounds. "T" stands for trace. This could vary from less than 1 carbo-cal to several or more, but not enough to affect your diet.

Note: Columns five, six, and seven do not always add up to column three. This seems on the face of it to be an error as there are only three types of calories. However, the differences crop up because some of the food item is not edible, as for instance the stalk ends in asparagus.

Two Ways to Use These Tables

There are two procedures for using these tables, depending on whether you are on the various high protein diets described in the previous chapters, or whether you are on the point system for precision protein dieting described in Chapter 11.

High, Higher, Highest Protein Diets. Select high protein foods that you like. Observe carbohydrate content. Under no condition select foods that will produce more than a daily total of 200 carbo-cals for the High Protein Diet, 100 carbo-cals for the Higher Protein Diet, or a trace for the Highest Protein (Crash) Diet.

Point System for Precision Protein Dieting. Select foods within the protein percentage requirements of the three diets. Then keep portions within the specified point limits.

Protein, Fat, Carbohydrate Calorie Content of Popular Foods

FOOD	Quantity	Food Energy Calories	Protein Percent	Protein Calorie	Fat Calorie	Carbo hydrate Calorie
MILK, CREAM, CHEESE, RELATED PRODUCTS						
Milk, Cow's						
fluid, non-fat (skim)	1 Cup	90	40	36	T	5
Buttermilk, cultured from skim milk	1 "	90	40	36	T	5
Dry, non-fat, instant	1 "	250	40	100	T	14
Cow's, fluid, whole (3.5% fat)	1 "	160	22	36		4
Evaporated, unsweetened, undiluted	1 "	345	21	72	180	9
Dry, whole	1 "	515	21	108	252	15
Milk, Goat's: fluid, whole	1 "	165	19	32	90	4
Condensed, sweetened, undiluted	1 "	980	10	100	243	64
Cream:						
Half-and-Half (cream and milk)	1 "	325	10	32	252	4
Light, coffee or table	1 "	505	6	28	441	4
Whipping, unwhipped, (volume about double when whipped)						
Light	1 "	715	3	24	675	3
Heavy	1 "	840	2	20	801	2

FOOD	Quantity	Food Energy Calories	Protein Percent	Protein Cal	Fat or	Carbo-hydrate ies
Cheese:						
Cottage Cheese, uncreamed, from skim milk	1 oz.	195	78	152	9	24
Cottage Cheese, creamed, from skim milk	1 "	240	52	124	81	28
Swiss Cheese, domestic	1 "	105	30	32	72	4
Cheddar, process	1 "	105	26	28	81	4
Cheese foods, Cheddar	1 "	90	26	24	63	8
Cheddar or American:						
Grated	1 cup	445	25	112	324	8
Ungrated	1 in. cube	70	22	16	45	T
Blue or Roquefort type	1 oz.	105	20	24	81	4
Cream Cheese	1 "	105	7	8	99	4
Milk Beverages:						
Malted Milk	1 cup	280	18	52	108	128
Chocolate flavored milk drink, (made with skim milk)	1 "	190	16	32	54	108
Cocoa	1 "	235	15	36	99	104
EGGS						
White of egg, raw	1 white	15	106	16	T	T
Boiled, shell removed	2 eggs	160	33	52	108	4
Raw, Whole, without shell	1 egg	80	30	24	54	T
Scrambled, with milk and fat	1 "	110	25	28	72	4
Yolk	1 yolk	60	20	12	45	T
MEAT, POULTRY, FISH, SHELLFISH, RELATED PRODUCTS						
Beef, trimmed to retail basis:						
Roast, oven-cooked, no liquid added						
Lean only	1.8 oz.	125	77	56	63	0
Heart, beef, lean, braised	3 "	160	68	108	45	4
Beef dried or chipped	2 "	115	66	76	36	0
Steak, broiled:						
Lean only	2.4 "	130	65	84	36	0
Relatively fat, such as sirloin:						
Lean only	2 "	115	63	72	36	0
Cuts, braised, simmered, or pot-roasted:						
Lean only	2.5 "	140	63	88	45	0
Roast, oven-cooked, no liquid added:						
Relatively lean, such as heel of round:						
Lean only	2.7 "	125	62	96	27	0
Lamb, trimmed to retail basis, cooked:						
Leg, roasted,						
Lean only	2.5 "	130	62	80	45	0
Beef, Roast oven-cooked, no liquid added,						
Relatively lean, such as heel of round:						
Lean and fat	3 "	165	61	100	63	0
Lamb, Chop, thick, with bone	1 chop					
Lean only	2.6 oz.	140	60	84	54	0
Pork, fresh, trimmed to retail basis, cooked:						
Cuts, simmered:						
Lean only	2.2 "	135	53	72	54	0
Lamb, trimmed to retail basis, cooked:						
Shoulder, roasted:						
Lean only	2.3 "	130	52	68	54	0
Hamburger, (ground beef), broiled:						
Lean	3 "	185	50	92	90	0
Veal, cooked:						
Cutlet, without bone, broiled	3 "	185	49	92	81	0
Corned Beef, canned	3 oz.	185	47	88	90	0
Steak, broiled: Lean and fat	3 "	220	46	96	117	0
Roast, oven-cooked, no liquid added:						
Relatively fat, such as rib:						

FOOD	Quantity	Food Energy Calories	Protein Percent	Protein Calories	Fat Calories	Carbohydrate Calories
Lean only	1.8 oz.	125	45	56	63	0
Beef, trimmed to retail basis, cooked:						
Cuts braised, simmered, or pot-roasted:						
Lean and fat	3 "	245	38	92	144	0
Lamb, trimmed to retail basis, cooked:						
Leg, roasted:						
Lean and fat	3 "	235	37	88	144	0
Hamburger (ground beef), broiled:						
Regular	3 "	245	34	84	153	0
Tongue, beef, braised	3 "	210	34	72	126	0
Pork, cured, cooked:						
Ham, light cure, lean and fat, roasted	3 "	245	29	72	171	0
Roast, oven-cooked, no liquid added:						
Lean and fat	3 "	310	27	84	216	0
Lamb, trimmed to retail basis, cooked:						
Chop, thick, with bone,						
1 chop, broiled	4.8 "	400	25	100	297	0
Lean and fat	4.0 "	400	25	100	297	0
Shoulder, roasted:						
Lean and fat	3 "	285	25	72	207	0
Pork, fresh, trimmed to retail basis, cooked:						
Chop, thick, with bone,						
1 chop,	3.5 "	260	25	64	189	0
Lean and fat	2.3 "	260	25	64	189	0
Cuts, simmered:						
Lean and fat	3 "	320	25	80	236	0
Steak, broiled:						
Relatively fat, such as sirloin:						
Lean and fat	3 "	330	24	80	243	0
Bacon, broiled or fried, crisp	2 slices	100	20	20	72	4
Chicken, cooked:						
Flesh only, broiled	3 oz.	115	70	80	27	0
Breast, fried, ½ breast:						
With bone	3.3 "	155	65	100	45	4
Flesh and skin only	2.7 "	155	65	100	45	4
Drumstick, fried:						
With bone,	2.1 "	90	53	48	36	0
Flesh and skin only	1.3 "	90	53	48	36	0
Chicken, canned, boneless	3 "	170	42	72	90	0
Fish and shellfish:						
Shrimp, canned, meat only	3 "	100	84	84	9	4
Crabmeat, canned	3 "	85	71	60	18	4
Clams:						
Raw, meat only	3 "	65	68	44	9	8
Bluefish, baked or broiled	3 "	135	65	88	36	0
Swordfish, broiled with butter or margarine	3 "	150	64	96	45	0
Clams:						
Canned, solids and liquid	3 "	45	62	28	9	8
Salmon, pink, canned	3 "	120	56	68	45	0
Tuna, canned in oil, drained	3 "	170	56	96	63	0
Oysters, meat only:						
Raw, 13-19 medium selects	1 cup	160	50	80	36	32
Haddock, fried	3 oz.	140	48	68	45	20
Shad, baked	3 "	170	47	80	90	0
Mackerel:						
Canned, Pacific, solids and liquid	3 "	155	46	72	81	0
Sardines, Atlantic, canned in oil, drained	3 "	175	46	80	81	0
Fish sticks, breaded, cooked, frozen; stick, 3.8 by 1.0 by 0.5 inch	8 "	400	38	152	180	60
Mackerel:						
Broiled, Atlantic	3 "	200	38	76	117	0
Ocean perch, breaded (egg and breadcrumbs), fried	3 "	195	33	64	99	24

FOOD	Quantity	Food Energy Calories	Protein Percent	Protein Calories	Fat Calories	Carbo-hydrates
Oyster stew, 1 part oysters to 3 parts milk by volume, 3 to 4 oysters	1 cup	200	22	44	108	44
Related Products:						
Beef, canned:						
Corned beef	3 oz.	185	48	88	90	0
Luncheon meat:						
Boiled ham, sliced	2 "	135	33	44	90	0
Chile con carne, canned:						
With beans	1 cup	335	23	76	135	120
Without beans	1 cup	510	20	104	342	60
Poultry potpie (based on chicken potpie).						
Individual pie, 4 ¼ inch diameter, weight before baking about 8 oz.	1 pie	535	17	92	279	168
Sausage:						
Bologna, slice, 4.1 by 0.1"	8 slices	690	17	108	558	8
Frankfurter, cooked	1	155	15	24	126	4
Pork, links or patty, cooked	4 oz.	540	15	84	450	0

MATURE DRY BEANS AND PEAS, NUTS, PEANUTS: RELATED PRODUCTS

FOOD	Quantity	Food Energy Calories	Protein Percent	Protein Calories	Fat Calories	Carbo-hydrates
Peas, split, dry, cooked	1 cup	290	28	80	9	208
Cowpeas or blackeye peas, dry, cooked	1 cup	190	27	52	9	136
Beans, dry:						
Common varieties, such as Great Northern, navy, and others, canned:						
Red	1 cup	230	26	60	9	168
Lima, cooked	1 cup	260	24	64	9	192
White, with tomato sauce:						
with pork	1 cup	320	20	64	63	200
without pork	1 cup	310	20	64	9	240
Peanuts, roasted, salted:						
Halves	1 cup	840	17	148	648	108
Peanut butter	1 tbs.	95	17	16	72	12
Peanuts, roasted, salted:						
Chopped	1 tbs.	55	15	8	36	8
Walnuts, shelled:						
Black or native, chopped	1 cup	790	13	104	675	76
Almonds, shelled	1 cup	850	12	104	693	112
Cashew nuts, roasted	1 cup	760	12	92	558	160
English or Persian:						
Halves	1 cup	650	9	60	576	64
Brazil nuts	1 cup	915	8	80	846	60
Pecans:						
Chopped	1 tbs.	50	8	4	45	4
English or Persian						
Chopped	1 tbs.	50	8	4	45	4
Pecans:						
Halves	1 cup	740	5	40	693	64
Coconut:						
Fresh, shredded	1 cup	335	3	12	306	36
Dried, shredded, sweetened	1 cup	340	2	8	216	132

VEGETABLES AND VEGETABLE PRODUCTS

FOOD	Quantity	Food Energy Calories	Protein Percent	Protein Calories	Fat Calories	Carbo-hydrates
Sprouts, raw:						
Soybean	1 cup	40	60	24	18	16
Kale, leaves including stems, cooked	1 cup	30	53	16	9	16
Broccoli spears, cooked	1 cup	40	50	20	0	28
Spinach:						
Cooked	1 cup	20	50	20	9	24
Cauliflower, cooked, flowerbuds	1 cup	25	48	12	0	20
Turnip greens: Cooked, in large amount of water, long time	1 cup	25	48	12	0	20
Asparagus: Cooked, cut spears	1 cup	35	45	16	0	24
Brussels sprouts, cooked	1 cup	45	44	20	0	28

FOOD	Quantity	Food Energy Calories	Protein Percent	Protein Calories	Fat Calories	Carbohydrate Calories
Spinach: Canned, drained solids	1 cup	45	44	20	9	24
Cabbage, spoon (or pakchoi), cooked.	1 cup	20	40	8	0	16
Asparagus: Canned spears, medium:						
Green	6 spears	20	40	8	0	12
Bleached	6 spears	20	40	8	0	16
Endive, curly (including escarole).	2 oz.	10	40	4	0	8
Lettuce, raw: Butterhead, as Boston types; head,						
4-inch diameter	1 head	30	40	12	0	24
Looseleaf, or bunching varieties, leaves	2 large	10	40	4	0	8
Spinach: Canned, strained or chopped (baby food).	1 oz.	10	40	4	0	8
Sprouts, raw: Mung bean	1 cup	30	40	12	0	24
Turnip greens: Cooked: In small amount of water,						
short time	1 cup	30	40	12	0	20
Collards, cooked	1 cup	55	36	20	9	36
Mustard greens, cooked	1 cup	35	34	12	9	24
Okra, cooked, pod 3 by 5/8 inch	8 pods	25	32	8	0	20
Peas, green, cooked	1 cup	115	31	36	9	76
Cowpeas, cooked, immature seeds	1 cup	175	30	52	9	116
Turnip greens, canned, solids and liquid	1 cup	40	30	12	9	28
Beans:						
Lima, immaturè, cooked	1 cup	180	27	48	9	128
Snap, green: Cooked: In small amount of water,						
short time	1 cup	30	27	8	0	28
Celery, raw: Pieces, diced	1 cup	15	27	4	0	16
Lettuce, raw: Crisphead, as Iceberg; head, 4 3/4 inch						
diameter	1 head	60	27	16	0	52
Peas, green: Canned, strained (baby food)	1 oz.	15	27	4	0	12
Peppers, sweet: Raw, medium, about 6 per pound:						
Green pod without stem and seeds	1 pod	15	27	4	0	12
Squash, Cooked: Summer, diced	1 cup	30	27	8	0	28
Beans, Snap, green, Cooked: In large amount of						
water, long time	1 cup	30	26	8	0	28
Cabbage: Cooked: In large amount of water, long time	1 cup	30	26	8	0	28
Cabbage, celery or Chinese: Raw, leaves and stalk,						
1 inch pieces	1 cup	15	26	4	0	12
Dandelion greens, cooked	1 cup	60	26	16	9	48
Cabbage, Cooked: In small amount of water,						
short time	1 cup	35	23	8	0	28
Peas, green: Canned, solids and liquid	1 cup	165	22	36	9	124
Tomatoes: Raw, medium 2 by 2½ inches, about 3 per						
pound	1 tomato	35	22	8	0	28
Carrots: Raw: Whole, 5½ by 1 inch, (25 thin strips).	1 carrot	20	20	4	0	20
Onions:						
Mature:						
Raw, onion 2½ inch diameter	1 onion	40	20	8	0	40
Cooked	1 cup	60	20	12	0	56
Young green, small, without tops	6 onions	20	20	4	0	20
Peppers, sweet:						
Red pod without stem and seeds	1 pod	20	20	4	0	16
Beans, Snap, green, Canned: Solids and liquid	1 cup	45	18	8	0	40
Sauerkraut, canned, solids and liquid	1 cup	45	18	8	0	36
Tomato juice, canned	1 cup	45	18	8	0	40
Corn, sweet: Cooked: ear 5 by 1 3/4 inches	1 ear	70	17	12	9	64
Beets, cooked, diced	1 cup	50	16	8	0	48
Peppers, hot, red, without seeds, diced (ground chili						
powder, added seasonings).	1 tbs.	50	16	8	18	32
Tomatoes: Canned	1 cup	50	16	8	0	40
Cucumbers, 10-ounce; 7½ by about 2 inches: Raw, pared	1 cuc.	30	13	4	0	28
Potatoes, medium (about 3 per pound raw):						
Baked, peeled after baking.	1 pot.	90	13	12	0	84
Mashed: Milk added	1 cup	125	13	16	9	100
Corn, sweet: Canned, solids and liquid	1 cup	170	12	20	18	160
Squash: Cooked: Winter, baked, mashed	1 cup	130	12	16	9	128

FOOD	Quantity	Food Energy Calories	Protein Percent	Protein C	Fat a l o r	Carbo-hydrate i e s
Potatoes, medium (about 3 per pound raw):						
Boiled: Peeled after boiling	1 pot.	105	11+	12	0	92
Turnips, cooked, diced	1 cup	35	11	4	0	32
Potatoes, medium (about 3 per pound raw):						
Peeled before boiling	1 pot.	80	10	8	0	72
Pumpkin, canned	1 cup	75	10	8	9	72
Carrots: Raw: Grated	1 cup	45	9	4	0	44
cooked: diced	1 cup	45	9	4	0	40
Potatoes, medium (about 3 per pound raw):						
Mashed: Milk and butter added	1 cup	185	9	16	72	96
Parsnips, cooked	1 cup	100	8	8	9	92
Sweet Potatoes: Canned, vacuum or solid	1 cup	235	7	16	0	216
Potatoes, medium (about 3 per pound raw):						
Frozen, heated	10 pcs.	125	6	8	45	76
French-fried, piece 2 by ½ by ½ inch: Cooked in deep fat	10 "	155	5	8	63	80
Sweet Potatoes: Cooked, medium, 5 by 2 inches, weight raw about 6 ounces:						
Baked, peeled after baking	1	155	5	8	9	144
Boiled, peeled after boiling	1	170	5	8	9	156
Cabbage, Raw: Coleslaw	1 cup	120	3	4	81	36
Potato chips, medium, 2-inch diameter	10 chips	115	3	4	72	40
Sweet Potatoes: Cooked, medium, 5 by 2 inches, weight raw about 6 ounces:						
Candied, 3½ by 2¼ inches	1	295	3	8	54	240
FRUITS AND FRUIT PRODUCTS						
Lemons, raw, medium, 2 1/5-inch diameter, size.	1 lemon	20	20	4	2	24
Oranges, raw: California, Navel (winter), 2 4/5-inch diameter	1 or.	60	13	8	0	64
Cherries: Raw, sweet with stems	1 cup	80	10	8	0	80
Pears, Canned, solids and liquid: Strained or chopped (baby food)	1 oz.	20	10	0	0	20
Tangerines, raw, medium, 2½-inch diameter, about 4 per pound	1	40	10	4	0	40
Blackberries, raw	1 cup	85	9	8	9	76
Apricots: Dried:						
Uncooked, 40 halves, small	1 cup	390	8	32	9	400
Cooked, unsweetened, fruit and liquid	1 cup	240	8	20	9	248
Apricots: Raw, about 12 per pound	3 ap.	55	7	4	0	56
Figs: Raw, small, 1½-inch diameter, about 12 per pound	1 fig	60	7	4	0	60
Grapefruit: Raw, medium, 4¼-inch diameter,						
White	1/2	55	7	4	0	56
Pink or red	1/2	60	7	4	0	60
Lemon Juice: Fresh	1 cup	60	7	4	2	80
Canned, unsweetened	1 cup	55	7	4	0	76
Orange juice: Fresh:						
California, Valencia (summer)	1 cup	115	7	8	9	104
Canned, unsweetened	1 cup	120	7	8	0	112
Strawberries: Raw, capped	1 cup	55	7	4	9	52
Watermelon, raw, wedge, 4 by 8 inches	1 wedge	115	7	8	9	108
Cantaloupes, raw, medium, 5-inch diameter, about 1 2/3 pound	1/2	60	6	4	0	56
Grapefruit: Canned, white:						
Water pack, solids and liquid	1 cup	70	6	4	0	72
Grapes, raw: American type (slip skin), such as Concord, Delaware, Niagara, Catawba, and Scuppernong	1 cup	65	6	4	9	60
Lime juice:						
Fresh	1 cup	65	6	4	0	88
Canned	1 cup	65	6	4	0	88
Orange juice:						
Frozen concentrate: Undiluted, can 6 fluid ounces	1 can	330	6	20	0	320
Dehydrated: Crystals, can, net weight 4 ounces	1 can	430	6	24	18	400
Papayas, raw, ½-inch	1 cup	70	6	4	0	72
Peaches: Raw, Sliced	1 cup	65	6	4	0	64

FOOD	Quantity	Food Energy Calories	Protein Percent	Protein Calories	Fat Calories	Carbohydrate Calories
Prunes, dried, "softenized," medium: Uncooked	4	70	6	4	0	72
Raspberries, red: Raw	1 cup	70	6	4	9	68
Apple brown betty	1 cup	345	5	16	72	272
Avocados, raw: California varieties, mainly Fuerte:						
½-inch cubes	1 cup	260	5	12	234	36
Florida varieties: 13-oz.	1/2	160	5	8	126	44
Bananas, raw, 6 by 1½ inches, about 3 per pound	1 ban.	85	5	4	0	92
Blueberries, raw	1 cup	85	5	4	9	84
Grapefruit: Raw sections, white	1 cup	75	5	4	0	80
Grapefruit juice: Frozen, concentrate, unsweetened:						
Undiluted, can, 6 fluid oz.	1 can	300	5	16	9	288
Dehydrated: Crystals, can, net weight 4 oz.	1 can	430	5	20	9	412
Oranges, raw: Florida, all varieties, 3-inch diameter	1	75	5	4	0	76
Orange and grapefruit juice:						
Frozen concentrate:						
Undiluted, can, 6 fluid oz.	1 can	325	5	16	9	312
Diluted with 3 parts water	1 cup	110	5	4	0	104
Peaches: Dried: Cooked, unsweetened, 10-12 halves and 6 tablespoons liquid	1 cup	220	5	12	9	232
Persimmons, Japanese or kaki, raw, seedless, 2½-inch diameter	1	75	5	4	0	80
Pineapple: Raw, diced	1 cup	75	5	4	0	76
Tangerine juice: Frozen concentrate: Undiluted, can, 6 fluid ounces	1 can	340	5	16	9	320
Apricots: Canned in heavy sirup:						
Halves and sirup	1 cup	220	4	8	0	228
Halves (medium) and sirup	2 tbs.	105	4	4	0	108
Avocados, raw: California varieties, mainly Fuerte:						
10-ounce avocado, about 3½ by 4¼ inches, peeled, pitted	1/2	185	4	8	162	24
Florida varieties: 1/2-inch cubes	1 cup	195	4	8	153	52
Figs: Raw, small, 1½-inch diameter, about 12 per pound	3 figs	90	4	4	92	
Grapefruit juice: Fresh	1 cup	95	4	4		92
Canned, white: Unsweetened	1 cup	100	4	4	96	
Diluted with 3 parts water	1 cup	100	4	4	2	96
Prepared with water	1 cup	100	4	4	2	96
Grapes, raw: European type, (adherent skin), such as Malaga, Muscat, Thompson Seedless, Emperor, and Flame Tokay	1 cup	95	4	4	2	100
Orange juice: Fresh						
Florida varieties: Early and mid-season	1 cup	100	4	4	0	92
Late season, Valencia	1 cup	110	4	4	0	104
Orange juice: Frozen concentrate: Diluted with 3 parts water, by volume	1 cup	110	4	4	0	108
Orange and grapefruit juice: Frozen concentrate: Diluted with 3 parts water, by volume	1 cup	110	4	4	0	104
Peaches: Dried, uncooked	1 cup	420	4	20	9	436
Pears: Raw, 3 by 2½-inch diameter	1 pear	100	4	4	9	100
Tangerine juice						
Canned, unsweetened	1 cup	105	4	4	0	100
Frozen concentrate: Diluted with 3 parts water, by volume	1 cup	115	4	4	0	108
Apricot nectar, canned	1 cup	140	3	4	0	144
Cherries: Canned, red, sour, pitted, heavy sirup	1 cup	230	3	8	9	236
Dates, domestic, natural and dry, pitted, cut	1 cup	490	3	16	9	520
Grapefruit juice:						
Canned, white:						
Sweetened	1 cup	130	3	4	0	128
Frozen, concentrate, sweetened:						
Undiluted can, 6 fluid oz.	1 can	350	3	12	9	340
Diluted with 3 parts water, by volume	1 cup	115	3	4	2	112
Pears, Canned, solids and liquid: Water pack	1 cup	80	3	0	0	80
Pear nectar, canned	1 cup	130	3	4	0	132
Pineapple juice, canned	1 cup	135	3	4	0	136

Protein, Fat, Carbohydrate Calorie Content of Popular Foods *(cont.)*

FOOD	Quantity	Food Energy Calories	Protein Percent	Protein Calories	Fat Calories	Carbohydrate Calories
Prunes, dried, "softenized," medium:						
Cooked, unsweetened, 17-18 prunes and 1/3 cup liquid	1 cup	295	3	8	9	312
Raisins, dried	1 cup	460	3	16	0	496
Raspberries, red: Frozen, 10-oz. carton, not thawed	1 car.	275	3	8	0	280
Tangerine juice: Frozen concentrate: Diluted with 3 parts water, by volume	1 cup	115	3	4	0	108
Applesauce, canned: Sweetened	1 cup	230	2	4	0	160
Fruit cocktail, canned in heavy sirup, solids and liquid	1 cup	195	2	4	9	200
Grapefruit: Canned, white: Sirup pack, solids and liquid.	1 cup	175	2	4	0	176
Grape juice, bottled or canned	1 cup	165	2	4	2	168
Lemon juice: Lemonade concentrate, frozen, sweetened: Diluted with 4 1/3 parts water, by volume	1 cup	110	2	0	0	112
Peaches: Canned, yellow-fleshed, solids and liquid: Sirup pack, heavy:						
Halves or slices	1 cup	200	2	4	0	208
Frozen, Can, 16 ounces, not thawed	1 can	400	2	8	0	412
Pears, Canned, solids and liquid: Sirup pack, heavy:						
Halves or slices	1 cup	195	2	4	9	200
Pineapple:	1 cup	195	2	4	0	200
Crushed	2 small or					
Sliced, slices and juice,	1 lg. and 2 tbs. juice	90	2	0	0	96
Plums, all except prunes:						
Canned, sirup pack (Italian prunes): Plums (with pits) and juice	1 cup	204	2	4	0	212
Prune juice, canned	1 cup	200	2	4	0	196
Strawberries: Frozen, 16-oz. can, not thawed.	1 can	495	2	8	9	504
Peaches: Raw, Whole, medium, 2-inch diameter, about 4 per pound	1 peach	35	1	4	0	40
Frozen: Carton, 12 ounces, not thawed	1 car.	300	1	4	0	308
Rhubarb, cooked, sugar added	1 cup	385	1	4	0	392
Strawberries: Frozen, 10-ounce carton, not thawed.	1 car.	310	1	4	9	316
Apples, raw, medium, 2½-inch diameter, about 3 per pound	1 apple	70	T	0	0	72
Apple juice, bottled or canned.	1 cup	120	T	0	0	120
Applesauce and apricots, canned, strained or junior (baby food)	1 oz.	25	T	0	0	24
Cranberry juice cocktail, canned.	1 cup	160	T	0	0	164
Cranberry sauce, sweetened, canned, strained.	1 cup	405	T	0	9	416
Lemonade concentrate, frozen, sweetened: Undiluted, can, 6 fluid ounces	1 can	430	T	0	0	448
Limeade concentrate, frozen, sweetened:						
Undiluted, can, 6 fluid oz.	1 can	410	T	0	0	432
Diluted with 4 1/3 parts water, by volume	1 cup	105	T	0	0	108
Peaches: Canned, yellow-fleshed, solids and liquid: Sirup pack, heavy: Halves (medium and sirup)	2 hal. and 2 tbs. sirup	90	T	0	0	96
Strained or chopped (baby food)	1 oz.	25	T	0	0	24
Peach nectar, canned	1 cup	120	T	0	0	124
Pears, Canned, solids and liquid: Sirup pack, heavy: Halves (medium) and sirup	2 halves and 2 tbs. sirup	90	T	0	0	92
Plums, all except prunes: Raw, 2-inch diameter, about 2 oz.	1 plum	25	T	0	0	28
Canned, sirup pack (Italian prunes): Plums (without pits) and juice	3 plums and 2 tbs. juice	100	T	0	0	104

GRAIN PRODUCTS

FOOD	Quantity	Food Energy Calories	Protein Percent	Protein Calories	Fat Calories	Carbohydrate Calories
Wheat germ, crude, commercially milled	1 cup	245	29	72	63	128
Spaghetti with meat balls in tomato sauce (home recipe).	1 cup	335	23	76	108	156

117

FOOD	Quantity	Food Energy Calories	Protein Percent	Protein Calories	Fat Calories	Carbohydrates
Rye wafers, whole-grain, 1 7/8 by 3½ inches	2 wafers	45	18	8	0	40
Whole-wheat bread, made with 2% nonfat dry milk:						
Loaf, 1-pound, 20 slices	1 loaf	1105	17	196	126	864
Wheat flours: Whole-wheat, from hard wheats, stirred	1 cup	64	16	18	16	340
Pumpernickel, loaf, 1 pound	1 loaf	1115	15	164	45	964
Macaroni (enriched) and cheese, baked	1 cup	470	15	72	216	176
Oatmeal or rolled oats, regular or quickcooking, cooked.	1 cup	130	15	20	18	92
Pizza (cheese); 5½-inch sector; 1/8 of 14-inch-diameter pie	1 sec.	185	15	28	54	108
Bran flakes (40% bran) added thiamine	1 oz.	85	14	12	9	92
Noodles (egg noodles), cooked: Enriched	1 cup	200	14	28	18	148
Unenriched	1 cup	200	14	28	18	148
Buckwheat (buckwheat pancake mix, made with egg and milk).	1 cake	55	14	8	18	24
Spaghetti in tomato sauce with cheese (home recipe).	1 cup	260	14	36	81	148
Cracked-wheat bread: Loaf, 1-lb. 20 slices	1 loaf	1190	13	156	90	944
Italian bread:						
Enriched, 1-pound loaf	1 loaf	1250	13	164	36	1024
Unenriched, 1-pound loaf	1 loaf	1250	13	164	36	1024
White bread, enriched: 1 to 2 percent non-fat dry milk:						
Loaf, 1-pound, 20 slices 3 to 4 percent non-fat dry milk:	1 loaf	1225	13	156	135	916
Loaf, 1-pound 5 to 6 percent non-fat dry milk:	1 loaf	1225	13	156	135	916
Loaf, 1-pound.	1 loaf	1245	13	164	153	912
White Bread, unenriched:						
1 to 2 percent non-fat dry milk:						
Loaf, 1 pound, 20 slices	1 loaf	1225	13	156	135	916
3 to 4 percent non-fat dry milk:						
Loaf, 1 pound	1 loaf	1225	13	156	135	916
5 to 6 percent non-fat dry milk:						
Loaf, 1 pound, 20 slices	1 loaf	1245	13	164	153	912
Bread crumbs, dry, grated	1 cup	345	13	44	36	260
Macaroni, cooked:						
Enriched:						
Cooked, firm stage	1 cup	190	13	24	9	156
Cooked until tender	1 cup	155	13	20	9	128
Unenriched:						
Cooked, firm stage	1 cup	190	13	24	9	156
Cooked until tender	1 cup	155	13	20	9	128
Pancakes (griddlecakes), 4-inch diameter: Wheat, enriched flour (home recipe).	1 cake	60	13	8	18	36
Spaghetti:						
Cooked, tender stage (14-20 min)						
Enriched	1 cup	155	13	20	9	128
Unenriched	1 cup	155	13	20	9	128
Waffles, with enriched flour, ½ by 4½ by 5½ inches	1 waffle	210	13	28	63	112
Breads:						
Boston brown bread, slice, 3 by 3/4 inch	1 slice	100	12	12	9	88
French or Vienna bread:						
Enriched, 1-pound loaf	1 loaf	1315	12	164	126	1004
Unenriched, 1 pound loaf	1 loaf	1315	12	164	126	1004
Farina, regular, enriched, cooked	1 cup	100	12	12	0	84
Rolls:						
Hard, round; 12 per 22 ounces	1 roll	160	12	20	18	124
Sweet, pan; 12 per 18 ounces	1 roll	135	12	16	36	84
Wheat, shredded, plain (long, round, or bitesize)	1 oz.	100	12	12	9	92
Wheatflakes, with added nutrients	1 oz.	100	12	12	0	92
Wheat flours: All purpose or family flour:						
Enriched, sifted	1 cup	400	12	48	9	336
Unenriched, sifted	1 cup	400	12	48	9	336
Cakes: Angelfood cake; sector, 2-inch (1/12 of 8-inch diameter cake)	1 sec.	110	11	12	0	96
Saltines, 2 inches square	2	35	11	4	9	24
Muffins, with enriched white flour; muffin, 2 3/4-inch diameter.	1 muf.	140	11	16	45	80

FOOD	Quantity	Food Energy Calories	Protein Percent	Protein Calories	Fat Calories	Carbohydrate Calories
Pies (piecrust made with unenriched flour): sector, 4-inch, 1/7 of 9-inch-diameter pie:						
Custard	1 sec.	280	11	32	126	120
Wheat, rolled; cooked	1 cup	175	11	20	9	160
Raisin bread: Loaf, 1-pound, 20 slices	1 loaf	1190	10	120	117	972
Sponge cake; sector, 2-inch (1/12 of 8-inch diameter cake)	1 sec.	120	10	12	18	88
Corn grits, degermed, cooked:						
Enriched	1 cup	120	10	12	0	108
Unenriched	1 cup	120	10	12	0	108
Cornmeal, white or yellow, dry:						
Whole ground, unbolted	1 cup	420	10	44	45	348
Rolls: Plain, pan; 12 per 16 ounces:						
Enriched	1 roll	115	10	12	18	80
Unenriched	1 roll	115	10	12	18	80
Barley, pearled, light, uncooked	1 cup	710	9	68	18	640
Biscuits, baking powder with enriched flour, 2½-inch diameter	1 bis.	140	9	12	54	68
Oyster crackers	10 crac.	45	9	4	9	28
Cracker meal	1 tbs.	45	9	4	9	28
Rice, white (fully milled or polished), enriched, cooked:						
Long grain, parboiled	1 cup	185	9	16	0	164
Wheat flours: Cake or pastry flour, sifted	1 cup	365	9	32	9	316
Cornmeal, white or yellow, dry: Degermed, enriched	1 cup	525	8	44	18	456
Corn muffins, made with enriched degermed cornmeal and enriched flour; muffin, 2 3/4-inch dia.	1 muf.	150	8	12	45	92
Soda Cracker, 2½-inch square	2 crac.	50	8	4	9	32
Wheat, puffed: With added nutrients, with sugar and honey	1 oz.	105	8	8	9	100
Cookies: Fig bars, small	1	55	7	4	9	48
Corn, rice and wheat flakes, mixed, added nutrients	1 oz.	110	7	8	0	96
Corn flakes, added nutrients: Plain	1 oz.	110	7	8	0	96
Corn, shredded, added nutrients	1 oz.	110	7	8	0	100
Crackers: Graham, plain	4 sm. or 2 med.	55	7	4	9	40
Pumpkin Pie (Piecrust made with unenriched flour) sector 4-inch, 1/7 of 9-inch-diameter pie.	1 sec.	275	7	20	135	128
Rice, puffed, added nutrients (without salt)	1 cup	55	7	4	9	52
Rice flakes, added nutrients	1 cup	115	7	8	2	104
Wheat and malted barley flakes, with added nutrients	1 oz.	110	7	8	T	96
Plain cake and cupcakes, without icing: Cupcake 2 3/4-inch diameter	1	145	6	8	54	88
Pound cake, old-fashioned (equal weights, flour, sugar, fat, eggs); slice, 2 3/4-by-3-by-5/8 inch	1 slice	140	6	8	81	56
Popcorn, popped, with added oil and salt	1 cup	65	6	4	21	32
Rice, white (fully milled or polished), enriched, cooked:						
Common commercial varieties, all types	1 cup	185	6	12	0	164
Gingerbread (made with enriched flour); piece, 2 by 2 by 2 in.	1 piece	175	5	8	54	116
Piecrust, plain, baked:						
Enriched flour:						
Lower crust, 9-inch shell	1 cru.	675	5	32	405	236
Double crust, 9-inch pie	1 d/c.	1350	5	64	810	472
Unenriched flour:						
Lower crust, 9-inch shell	1 cru.	675	5	32	405	236
Double crust, 9-inch pie	1 d/c.	1350	5	64	810	472
Pies (piecrust made with unenriched flour); sector, 4-inch, 1/7 of 9-inch diameter pie:						
Cherry	1 sec.	355	5	16	135	208
Lemon meringue	1 sec.	305	5	16	108	180
Plain cake and cupcakes, without icing:						
Piece, 3 by 2 by 1½ inches	1 piece	200	4	8	72	124
Plain cake and cupcakes, with chocolate icing:						
Sector, 2-inch (1/16 of 10-inch layer cake)	1 sec.	370	4	16	126	236
Cupcake, 2 3/4-inch diameter	1	185	4	8	63	120
Corn flakes, added nutrients, Sugar-covered	1 oz.	110	4	4	0	104

FOOD	Quantity	Food Energy Calories	Protein P cent	Protein C a l	Fat o r i	Carbo-hydrate e s
Corn, puffed, pre-sweetened, added nutrients	1 oz.	110	4	4	0	104
Fruitcake, dark (made with enriched flour) piece 2, by 2 by ½ in.	1 piece	115	3	4	45	72
Cookies: Plain and assorted, 3-inch diameter	1	120	3	4	45	72
Doughnuts, cake type	1	125	3	4	54	64
Pies, (piecrust made with unenriched flour); sector, 4-inch, 1/7 of 9-inch-diameter pie						
Apple Pie	1 sec.	345	3	12	135	204
Mince	1 sec.	365	3	12	144	224
Pretzels, small stick	5 sticks	20	T	0	0	16

FATS, OILS

FOOD	Quantity	Food Energy Calories	Protein P cent	Protein C a l	Fat o r i	Carbo-hydrate e s
Salad dressings:						
Home cooked, boiled	1 tbs.	30	13	4	18	12
Blue cheese	1 tbs.	80	5	4	72	4
Thousand Island	1 tbs.	75	3	0	12	8
Mayonnaise	1 tbs.	110	2	0	108	2
Butter, 4 sticks per pound:						
Sticks, 2	1 cup	1625	T	4	1656	4
Margarine, 4 sticks per pound:						
Sticks, 2	1 cup	1635	T	4	1656	4
Salad dressings:						
Commercial, mayonnaise type	1 tbs.	65	T	0	54	8
French	1 tbs.	60	T	0	54	12
Fats, cooking:						
Lard	1 cup	1985	0	0	1980	0
Vegetable fats	1 cup	1770	0	0	1800	0
Oils, salad or cooking:						
Corn .	1 tbs.	125	0	0	126	0
Cottonseed	1 tbs.	125	0	0	126	0
Olive	1 tbs.	125	0	0	126	0
Soybean	1 tbs.	125	0	0	126	0

SUGARS, SWEETS

FOOD	Quantity	Food Energy Calories	Protein P cent	Protein C a l	Fat o r i	Carbo-hydrate e s
Candy:						
Marshmallows	1 oz.	90	8	4	0	92
Chocolate, milk, plain	1 oz.	150	5	8	81	64
Chocolate sirup, thin type	1 tbs.	50	4	0	0	52
Jams and preserves	1 tbs.	55	4	0	0	56
Jellies:	1 tbs.	55	4	0	0	56
Candy:						
Caramels	1 oz.	115	3	4	27	88
Fudge, plain	1 oz.	115	3	4	27	84
Honey, strained or extracted	1 tbs.	65	3	0	0	68
Molasses, cane:						
Light (First extraction)	1 tbs.	50	0	0	0	52
Blackstrap (third extraction)	1 tbs.	45	0	0	0	44
Sirup, table blends (chiefly corn, light and dark)	1 tbs.	60	0	0	0	60
Sugars (cane or beet);						
Granulated	1 cup	770	0	0	0	796
Lump, 1 1/8 by 3/4 by 3/8	1 lump	25	0	0	0	24
Powdered, stirred before measuring	1 cup	495	0	0	0	508
Brown, firm-packed	1 cup	820	0	0	0	848

MISCELLANEOUS ITEMS

FOOD	Quantity	Food Energy Calories	Protein P cent	Protein C a l	Fat o r i	Carbo-hydrate e s
Gelatin, dry: Plain	1 tbs.	35	103	36	2	0
Bouillon cube, 5/8 inch	1 cube	5	80	4	0	?
Soups, canned; ready-to-serve (prepared with equal volume of water):						
Beef bouillon, broth, consommé	1 cup	30	67	20	0	12
Yeast:						
Baker's:						
Dry active	1 oz.	80	50	40	2	44
Compressed	1 oz.	25	48	12	2	12
Brewer's, dry, debittered	1 tbs.	25	48	12	2	12

FOOD	Quantity	Food Energy Calories	Protein Percent	Protein Calories	Fat Calories	Carbo hydrate Calories
Pickles, cucumber: Dill, large, 4 by 1 3/4 inches	1	15	26	4	2	12
Soups, canned; ready-to-serve (prepared with equal volume of water):						
Chicken noodle	1 cup	65	26	16	18	32
Beef noodle	1 cup	70	25	16	27	28
Bean with pork	1 cup	170	19	32	54	88
Minestrone	1 cup	105	19	20	27	56
Pea, green	1 cup	130	19	24	18	92
Vegetable with beef broth	1 cup	80	15	12	18	56
Olives, pickled:	4 med.					
Green	3 extra large or 2 giant	15	13	2	18	2
Ripe: Mission	3 small 2 large	15	13	2	18	2
Gelatin dessert, ready-to-eat: Plain	1 cup	140	11	16	0	136
Chili sauce (mainly tomatoes)	1 tbs.	20	10	2	0	16
Gelatin, dry: Dessert powder, 8-ounce package	½ cup	315	10	32	0	300
Soups, canned; ready-to-serve (prepared with equal volume of water):						
Clam chowder	1 cup	85	9	8	27	52
Tomato	1 cup	90	9	8	18	64
White sauce, medium	1 cup	430	9	40	297	92
Chocolate:						
Bitter or baking	1 oz.	145	8	12	135	32
Gelatin dessert, ready-to-eat: With fruit	1 cup	160	8	12	2	160
Pickles, cucumber: Sweet, 2 3/4 by 3/4 inches	1	30	7	2	2	28
Soups, canned; ready-to-serve (prepared with equal volume of water):						
Cream soup (mushroom)	1 cup	135	6	8	90	40
Beer (average 3.6 percent alcohol by weight).	1 cup	100	4	4	0	36
Starch (cornstarch)	1 cup	465	T	2	2	448
Tapioca, quick cooking, granulated, dry, stirred before measuring	1 cup	535	T	4	2	524
Vinegar	1 tbs;	2	0	0	0	4
Beverages, carbonated:						
Cola type	1 cup	95	0	0	0	96
Ginger ale	1 cup	70	0	0	0	72

7

THIRTY DAYS
OF PLEASURABLE DINING
AS YOU LOSE
POUND AFTER POUND ON
THE FAT DESTROYER DIET

Do you like shad roe? Flavored with parsley, tarragon, chervil, and chives, it is a connoisseur's treat.

How about roast duckling? Shall we have it tonight a l'orange or en vin?

Or are you rather a steak smothered in onions type, or a hamburger and hot dog plebeian?

Little matter. Whoever you are and whatever turns on your taste buds, there's a High Protein bill of fare and a Higher Protein bill of fare to keep you interested and delighted for day after day without repetition, hunger, or boredom.

No, not melba toast and carrot sticks, cottage cheese and celery stalks—these have become legend in conventional dietary circles because there are a limited number of low calorie foods. You have to eat the same foods day in and day out on low calorie diets.

But on High Protein diets, calories be damned. We are more interested in cutting out carbohydrates than in cutting down on calorie quantities.

122

Thank your lucky palate that there are no limits to high protein, fat burning foods.

When I make suggestions to my slenderizing clients, I like to include some imaginative selections to broaden their menu-making horizons.

One day, I mentioned to a middle-aged school teacher, on her first week of weight loss, that there was a sign in the local fish store offering frogs' legs.

"Oh," she gasped, "If I have to eat those I'll die."

No, dear reader, you don't have to eat frogs' legs, or veal kidneys, or tripe, or brains, or turtle steaks, or venison, or snails.

But just in case you relish any of these "exotic" foods, they are all on your High Protein, Higher Protein and Highest Protein programs.

They are the programs that say "yes."

They also say "yes" to the more everyday type of supermarket foods that are proteins. You can choose to prepare them plainly or you can fancy them up.

Fat Destroying High Protein Foods

If you want to refresh your memory as to the variety of high protein, no carbohydrate foods available for menu planning, check the 100 percent protein foods and no carbohydrate items listed on the calorie and percentage tables in Chapter 6. Since a carbohydrate-free food does not exclude fat, these acceptable items may not show 100 percent protein. So the key is the right-hand column (Carbohydrate Calories). Any item indicating 0 or T or a number preferably under five, and certainly under 10, is eligible.

But then, of these eligible items, you should favor those with the highest percent of protein and lowest percent of fat.

See list of High Protein Fat Destroying Foods on p. 124. It is in no way complete but offered simply as a memory jogger.

The list could be extended considerably, especially if all the different cuts and cooking methods were listed. Take beef. Again, this list is not complete, but enough to start your salivary glands flowing. (See list of Beef Cuts on p. 124):

Certainly, there are as many cuts of pork and lamb. There are also smoked and seasoned cuts, like bacon and corned beef.

High Protein Fat Destroying Foods

(Insignificant Carbohydrate Content)

Meat	Organ Meats	Shellfish	Poultry
Beef	Tripe	Lobster	Chicken
Lamb	Heart	Crab	Turkey
Pork	Liver	Oyster	Goose
Veal	Kidney	Bay Scallop	Duck
Rabbit	Tongue	Mussel	Squab
Venison	Brain	Clam	Guinea Hen
Sausage		Crayfish	Pheasant
Wursts			Quail

Fish		Cheese	Eggs
Trout	Pike	Camembert	(Cooking
Cod	Bluefish	Gorgonzola	Method)
Sole	Herring	Bel Paese	
Perch	White fish	Cheddar	Soft boiled
Smelts	Mackerel	Cream	Hard boiled
Halibut	Carp	Cottage	Shirred
Haddock	Porgy	Pot	Fried
Salmon	Pompano	American	Scrambled
Flounder	Shad	Swiss	Omelette
Tuna	Sardines	Gruyère	Poached
Finnan	Snapper	Mozzarella	Egg Nog
Haddie	Whiting	Roquefort	
Bass		Blue	
		Port Salut	
		Jack	
		Farmer's	
		Muenster	

Beef Cuts

(Not Including Organs)

Roast beef	Brisket of beef	Cube steak
Potted steak	T-bone steak	Rump steak
Barbequed steak	Filet mignon	Oxtail
Flank steak	Chopped steak	Sirloin steak
Short ribs	Beef frankfurters	Porterhouse steak
Beef stew	Chipped beef	Rib steak
Pot roast	Corned beef	

With several ways of preparing each cut, there are probably over 50 beef dishes, alone, that you can come up with.

And there are probably over one thousand ways to prepare all of the high protein fat destroying foods listed, not to speak of others not on the list.

Figuring three meals a day, that's still one whole year without repeating the same dish.

And you can eat all you want of each dish!

Do you see now why this "diet" is so successful? It's really not a diet at all. It's a slenderizing way of life.

Keys to Successful Thinning Menus

Variety makes for eating satisfaction.

We have a number of oral needs. Sometimes we are in the mood for something hot or something cold. We feel this type of oral need. But others are less obvious. Something bland or something spicy? Something crisp or something soft? Something wet or something dry? These are all oral choices that have subtle voices. Unless these voices are heard and acted on, they get loud and insistent.

It was recently reported in the press that smokers do indeed gain some weight when they become ex-smokers. Two doctors studied 500 telephone workers for some five years or more. They were men 40 to 60 years of age. Those who stopped smoking during the test gained an average of 11 pounds, while non-smokers inched up only two pounds. The cause: oral needs expressing themselves as hunger.

If you are on a conventional low calorie diet, you are so limited in your menus that a number of unsatisfied oral needs become very vociferous. In effect, they say, "Quit!"

The same is true for the Highest Protein (Crash) Diet. It takes guts to stay on it, and unwanted fat around your gut to motivate you.

So no menus are provided in this chapter for that diet. The sample menus in Chapter 5 should suffice to keep you on that straight and narrow path.

However, the High and Higher Protein Diets are not that

straight nor anywhere near that narrow. Thirty days of diversified menus are set forth on the pages ahead.

These suggest 90 meals out of a possible thousand or more. So don't limit yourself to these menus.

Do "your own thing."

There Are a Few Important Guidelines to Keep in Mind

Guideline #1. Keep a close watch on carbo-cals. They have a way of sneaking in. Exclude dishes from your menu, if they contain sugar, bread or bread crumbs, flour or starch.

It is better to use heavy cream to thicken a soup, gravy, or sauce than flour. And let a stew stew in its own natural juices.

Both diets call for one portion of vegetable, one of fruit, and one of salad. If a vegetable goes into a casserole, no other vegetable should be served that day. If you have fruit or juice for breakfast, no fruit that night for dessert.

However, you can be more lenient when it comes to salad. A few sprigs of parsley or watercress alongside that luncheon omelette should not be considered to preempt your dinner salad.

Guideline #2. Favor low fat foods. Given a choice, check the tables in this book for fat content. Pick the lower. Fat cuts your oral satisfaction down in half as it fills you up twice as fast as proteins with the same weight of food.

Guideline #3. Favor high nutritive foods. I have already talked about these: fresh, local, unprocessed, unrefined, unpolluted with preservatives and chemicals. Favor vegetables that are loaded with minerals and vitamins. The same for fruits. Favor high protein over low protein. Favor organic over chemically fertilized and sprayed. Include fish and organ meats in menu planning. Feed your body cells and you won't feel hungry as often.

Guideline #4. Diversify. Be adventuresome. Try new foods. Try new ways of preparing familiar foods.

Guideline #5. Plan ahead. It pays to work out your menus for a number of days ahead when you go shopping. A half of grapefruit left over from a dinner dessert should be used for the next morning's breakfast. And why buy a small roast when a larger one can serve for two meals, a lunch and a couple of in-between snacks.

Guideline #6. Respect your intuitive leanings but be discerning between natural needs and unnatural cravings. Why schedule mixed greens in the name of diversity when you just love green peppers.

An onion a day is what a 92-year old steelworker at the Bethlehem Steel plant in San Francisco credits for his superb fitness. He handles 20-pound steel bars as deftly as co-workers 30 years his junior and has no plans to retire. Can you imagine what he'd do if his wife put a tomato instead of an onion in his lunch box?

How to Use the 30 Days of Special Menus in This Book

In the pages ahead, there are menus for 30 days of diversified dining. On the left side of the page are the menus for the Standard High Protein Diet. On the right hand are changes for the Higher Protein Diet.

The Higher Protein Diet differs only in the reduction of some fats and some carbohydrates. I have been very conservative in selecting foods for the High Protein Diet so the gap between the two diets is somewhat narrowed.

Still, you will see that heavy cream in coffee and lemon in tea, while permitted in one, is not called for in the other. This is because it is presumed that the reason you are on the Higher is that you need a temporary boost to your weight loss to reach your goal.

Once you attain that goal, you can move across the page, from the right side to the left.

The High Protein Diet is a maintenance diet. That is, it not only destroys excess fat, it keeps it off. While you are on it to lose weight, you will be wise to be very strict in your observance of the carbohydrate limitations. Eat all you want of meat, fish, poultry, eggs, and cheese. But observe carbo-cal limitations to the letter.

When you reach your desired weight, you can add a fruit or a vegetable or an occasional dessert. But keep your eye on the scale. You may have to lower the carbo-cal boom on yourself once again.

You can skip around on the menu days, but within each day there is that day's requirements or limitations. So don't pick breakfast from the 18th day and dinner from the 17th day and place them on the same day or else the carbo-cals in a whole cantaloupe will have a chance to hang some weight on you.

Some days are rather festive. Like roast turkey on the 12th day. You can shuffle these around to suit your calendar. But note, too, that the leftovers are scheduled in subsequent days' menus.

It is presumed that you know how to handle common preparations or have basic recipe books in your kitchen. Special dishes are keyed to the recipes in the following chapter.

If You Must Have Desserts . . .

Did you ever eat in a Korean restaurant and at the end of the meal ask the waitress for a dessert? No way. Koreans don't require desserts. Japanese restaurants rarely offer a dessert. Chinese restaurants offer almond cookies or fortune cookies largely to please westerners; they might also have kumquats or pineapple.

Half the people of the world do not have the dessert habit. They are the slender people of the world. Korean doctors do not specialize in obesity—they would have empty offices. Nor do Korean authors write diet books. They would have empty stomachs.

It is the dessert half of the world that has a weight problem.

Still, there are ways to satisfy your propensity for desserts while losing weight on the Free Diet, High Protein Diet, and Higher Protein Diet. These are limited, but two doors are open:

1. Fruit can be had as a dinner dessert instead of for breakfast.
2. Eggs, cheese, cream, milk, and butter are excellent dessert ingredients.

Your breakfast orange, grapefruit, or tangerine makes an adequate dinner dessert. However, there are other fruits that you enjoy which can get by with certain precautions.

First, remember that you are exercising an iron-clad control over carbo-cals. Should you ease up on this control for even 50 carbo-cals, you take the fat destroying ability away from the proteins you ate that day. You can turn weight loss into weight gain.

Here are suggested guidelines for the distribution of carbo-cals on both the High and Higher Protein Diets.

Suggested Distribution of Carbo-cals

Diet	Salad	Vegetable	Fruit or Dessert
High Protein	40	60	100
Higher Protein	20	30	50

With a 100 carbo-cal allowance, there are hardly any fruits you need to worry about. Berries, melons, pears, peaches, and apples are certainly eligible, but . . . in the case of canned or frozen products, you must drain the sugary syrup and rinse.

With a 50 carbo-cal allowance, the portion must be watched carefully and certain fruits—bananas, pears, and cherries—are too high in carbo-cals even to consider.

Even taboo fruits can be considered eligible if you can combine a fraction of the fruit per portion with protein foods such as cheese or whipped cream. For instance, a banana blended with whipped cream can make a banana whip for two for a Higher Protein Diet dessert.

See the Non-Fruit Dessert Ideas on p. 130 for other dessert ideas for each diet with approximate carbo-cal content:

Note that while one scoop of ice cream makes the list, sherbet, or ice, does not due to the greater amounts of sugar used. This use of sugar in any of the above desserts, or other sweeteners such as honey, is where the carbo-cals mostly add up. Be extremely economical in your use of sweeteners; use synthetic diet sweeteners instead if you can.

Non-Fruit Dessert Ideas

(All portions ½ cup unless otherwise stated)

High Protein Diet		Higher Protein Diet	
(Approx. 100 Carbo-cal Limit)		(Approx. 50 Carbo-cal Limit)	
Ice Cream (one scoop)	75	Butterscotch Pudding	
Zabaglione (see recipes)	70	(½ cup sugar free)	40
Chocolate Blanc Mange	100	Baked Indian Pudding	50
Vanilla Blanc Mange	90	Junket	20
Butterscotch Pudding (1/3 cup)	80	Caramel Custard	50
Apple Snow	70	Floating Island	50
Bavarian Cream (see recipes)	100	Fruit-flavored Gelatin	
Vanilla Pudding	95	(4 oz.)	50
Rice Pudding	70		
Plus all those on Higher Protein Diet list			

GENERAL WARNING: When you put any of the desserts listed above on your menu, you do so at the expense of minerals and vitamins that you would otherwise benefit from in fruit. To do so frequently could starve the body of needed fat metabolizing nutrients. The use of vitamins and mineral supplements would then be advisable.

Your Best Desserts

Your best desserts are fresh fruit or cheese. You can even have both. You can have whipped cream on your fruit.

One precaution where cream is used for desserts; you might go easy that day in its use in coffee. The higher the protein percentage, the more weight you will lose. Protein percentage goes down as fat content goes up. No carbo-cal problem here, but fat contains double the energy and this can activate the storage process.

You don't need to eat a dessert if you have had a satisfying dinner. I would much rather see you have another portion of pot roast or another chicken leg or a second helping of salmon or a third.

Juices, Soups and Beverages

Liquids are often the "Trojan horse" of diets. They seem harmless enough but they can carry a carload of carbo-cals into your system quite unsuspectingly.

Fruit is on the Higher Protein Diet but not fruit juice. Before you can start to enjoy a glass of orange juice, you have exceeded the carbo-cals in an orange. Canned juices are usually injected with sugar. Even the frozen juice is sometimes. One wonders why it is necessary in the frozen variety, since its preservative aspect is not needed, but the legend on the frozen can usually explain it as required for quality or uniformity.

Juices with sugar added are taboo. Always read the juice label.

Even juices without sugar added must be kept under tight rein. A six-ounce can of frozen orange juice makes 24 ounces of juice with 320 carbo-cals dancing around in joyful expectation. A six-ounce glass brings fruition to the hopes of 25 percent of them. Eighty carbo-cals pour into your stomach looking for prote-cals to seduce.

What happens if you use an eight-ounce glass and fill it more than three-quarters full? I'm afraid that's it for the day, my friend.

I recommend that you use a standard paper cup for your juice—the five-ounce dispenser variety—and play it safe.

Of course, you can drink all the water you want. In fact, the higher the protein diet you are on, the more water is recommended. It seems to flush your system of the ketones and other by-products of fat destruction.

Beverages

Coffee and tea are on the menus that follow. So are diet sodas. This is not because I recommend them, but because they are a part of our culture and the lesser of a number of other evils that are our way of life.

A recent survey of heavy drinkers of coffee, that is, eight cups a day, showed that they were much more prone to heart problems than the non-drinkers and moderate coffee drinkers. Coffee is also known to play tricks with the pancreas where blood sugar is regulated.

Tea is a stimulant, but not as dimly regarded as coffee in health circles.

Colas contain caffeine. So if diet colas don't catch you the calorie way, they may be bad for you the cardiac way.

Diet sodas with low calorie synthetic sweeteners are themselves suspect in large doses. Just be forewarned that one day we may discover some unwanted long-range effects from imbibing these chemicalized sodas by the six pack.

Cyclamate causes cancer of the bladder in rats when consumed in very large quantities. Saccharin produces the same effects. The government is considering banning both.

However, nature herself may have come up with the answer. A soluble protein material with 3,000 times the sweetening power of an equal weight of sugar has been discovered in West Africa. Dr. James Morris and Dr. Robert Cagan of the Monell Chemical Senses Center at the University of Pennsylvania have isolated the material from a West African wild red berry with the Latin name Diocorephyllum Cumminsii. The name being given to the sugar substitute is Monellin, but it may be years before the West Africans raise crops to compete with sugar cane or before it is synthesized in the laboratory.

So meanwhile, we are back to water as your best beverage. But if you have to indulge in the others, do so in moderation.

Soups

Soups are limited to those made with meat extracts and those made with vegetable and cream. The latter take the place of the vegetable allowance for the day. However, beef bouillon or chicken broth are "free."

This Menu Permits You to Eat All You Want of the Fat Destroyer Foods

Limits are placed in your menu listings for juice, fruit, or vegetables and sometimes even salad.

But as you look over the breakfast menu and wonder how many eggs "scrambled eggs" call for per portion, forget it. Have one, two, or three. Or if you remember the good old days when four slices of bacon never brought a blink of the eye, the good old days are back.

All you want. That is the size of the bacon, eggs, sausage, and ham portions.

At lunch, feel like another hamburger patty? Go ahead. And don't spare the meat.

At dinner, when you slice into the roast lamb for a third time, you are not making a pig of yourself, you are making a slender, attractive person.

If snacks are protein, have a snack anytime you feel like it. Cook plenty of chicken parts or flank steak, so that cold chicken and cold steak are there waiting for you—instead of a handful of insidious potato chips or a treacherous piece of pie.

Cheeses make fine satisfying snacks and good desserts. Get to know the many varieties available, especially the unprocessed, natural varieties. Imported cheeses offer a world of tastes and textures.

There's no starvation ahead. Quite the contrary. There's endless feasting ahead as you slim down.

Bon appetit. Following is your 30-day eating program. Enjoy it!

30 DAY PROGRAM

HIGH PROTEIN DIET	HIGHER PROTEIN DIET

FIRST DAY

Breakfast

Tangerine Juice (6 oz.)	Tangerine
Eggs, fried	Same
Bacon	Same
Coffee, heavy cream	Coffee, black

Lunch

Hot Lobster Salad (see recipes)	Same
Tea, lemon wedge	Tea, plain

Dinner

Consommé, cup	Same
Roast Prime Ribs of Beef	Same
Watercress	Same
Assorted Cheese	None
Coffee, heavy cream	Coffee, black

HIGH PROTEIN DIET	HIGHER PROTEIN DIET
	Snack
Cold Roast Beef	Same

SECOND DAY

Breakfast

½ Cantaloupe	¼ Cantaloupe
Eggs, scrambled	Same
Coffee, heavy cream	Coffee, black

Lunch

Blended Soup (see recipes)	Hot Protein Broth (see recipes)
Camembert Cheese	Leftover Meat or Fish
Tea, lemon wedge	Tea, plain

Dinner

Liver and Bacon with Cabbage (see recipes)	Same
Gelatin Dessert (diet type)	Same
Coffee, heavy cream	Coffee, black

Snack

Cold Roast Beef	Same

THIRD DAY

Breakfast

Orange Juice (6 oz.)	Orange
Ham Steak	Same
Coffee, heavy cream	Coffee, black

Lunch

Mushroom Omelette	Same
Tea, lemon wedge	Tea, plain

Dinner

Shoulder Lamb Chops	Same
Large Mixed Green Salad with Dressing	Small Mixed Green Salad
Coffee, heavy cream	Coffee, black

Snack

Ham Slices	Same

FOURTH DAY

Breakfast

Grapefruit Juice, unsweetened (6 oz.)	Half Grapefruit

HIGH PROTEIN DIET

Link Sausages
Scrambled Eggs
Coffee, heavy cream

Ham and Cheese Slices
Diet Soda

Broiled Sirloin Steak
Brussels Sprouts, average portion
Coffee, heavy cream

Cold Steak

HIGHER PROTEIN DIET

Same
Same
Coffee, black

Lunch
Ham Slices
Same

Dinner
Same
Cauliflower, small portion
Coffee, black

Snack
Same

FIFTH DAY

Breakfast

Whole Orange
Creamed Chipped Beef
Coffee, heavy cream

Eggs Curry (see recipes)
Tea, lemon wedge

Hearty Halibut (see recipes)
Cauliflower, average portion
Mixed salad, dressing
Coffee, heavy cream

Cold Steak

Same
Same
Coffee, black

Lunch
Eggs in Hot Sauce (see recipes)
Tea, plain

Dinner
Savory Baked Halibut (see recipes)
Cauliflower, small portion
Same
Coffee, black

Snack
Same

SIXTH DAY

Breakfast

Bacon and Eggs, any style
Coffee, heavy cream

Hamburger Steak
Celery Salad (see recipes)
Diet Cola

Same
Coffee, black

Lunch
Same
Same
Same

HIGH PROTEIN DIET	HIGHER PROTEIN DIET

Dinner

Broiled Sweetbreads	Same
Eggplant Italienne (see recipes)	Plain Eggplant
Melon Melé (see recipes)	Same
Coffee, heavy cream	Coffee, black

Snack

| Cheese | Leftover Meat or Fish |

SEVENTH DAY

Breakfast

Melon Melé	Same
Ham and Eggs, any style	Same
Coffee, heavy cream	Coffee, black

Lunch

Marinated Mushroom Platter	Same
(see recipes)	Same
Tea, lemon wedge	Tea, plain

Dinner

Pacific Veal (see recipes)	Same
Lettuce, Bamboo Shoots, Watercress,	
Dressing	Same
Assorted Cheese	None
Coffee, heavy cream	Coffee, black

Snack

| Thai Tuna (see recipes) | Same |

EIGHTH DAY

Breakfast

Sliced Fresh Peach, heavy cream	Sliced Fresh Peach, medium
Soft Boiled Eggs	Same
Coffee, heavy cream	Coffee, black

Lunch

Thai Tuna (see recipes)	Same
Assorted Cheese	Leftover Meat or Fish
Tea, lemon wedge	Tea, plain

Dinner

| Salmon Paysanne (see recipes) | Broiled Yellow Perch (see recipes) |

HIGH PROTEIN DIET	HIGHER PROTEIN DIET
Asparagus	Same
Zabaglione (see recipes)	Same
Coffee, heavy cream	Coffee, black

Snack

Hard Boiled Egg(s)	Same

NINTH DAY

Breakfast

Berries, drain sugar, average portion	Berries, drain sugar, small portion
Omelette	Same
Coffee, heavy cream	Coffee, black

Lunch

Cold Salmon Paysanne (leftover)	Same
Watercress	Same
Tea, lemon wedge	Tea, plain

Dinner

Roast Leg of Lamb	Same
String Beans	Same
Assorted Cheeses	None
Coffee, heavy cream	Coffee, black

Snack

Cold Lamb Slices	Same

TENTH DAY

Breakfast

Orange Juice, 6 oz.	Medium Orange
Veal Kidneys, broiled	Same
Coffee, heavy cream	Coffee, black

Lunch

Reheated Lamb, natural gravy	Same
Cold String Beans	Same
Diet Soda	Same

Dinner

Chicken Palau (see recipes)	Broiled Chicken
Broccoli	Same
Coffee, heavy cream	Coffee, black

Snack

Cold Lamb Slices	Same

HIGH PROTEIN DIET	HIGHER PROTEIN DIET

ELEVENTH DAY

Breakfast

Fresh Pear, medium	Fresh Pear, small
Small Breakfast Steak	Same
Coffee, heavy cream	Coffee, black

Lunch

| Eggs En Gelée (see recipes) | Same |
| Tea, lemon wedge | Tea, plain |

Dinner

Broiled Calf's Liver	Same
Steamed Cabbage with Butter	Same
Diet Dessert	Same
Coffee, heavy cream	Coffee, black

Snack

| Leftover Eggs En Gelée | Same |

TWELFTH DAY

Breakfast

| Eggs and Link Sausage | Same |
| Coffee, heavy cream | Coffee, black |

Lunch

| Hamburger Patties with Melted Cheese | Hamburger Patties |
| Ice Coffee | Same |

Dinner

Roast Turkey	Same
Zucchini	Same
Mixed Green Salad	Same
Coffee, heavy cream	Coffee, black

Snack

| Apple, medium | Same |

THIRTEENTH DAY

Breakfast

Apple Juice, 4 oz.	Apple, medium
Chopped Turkey Liver	Same
Coffee, heavy cream	Coffee, black

Lunch

| Beef Bouillon, cup | Same |

HIGH PROTEIN DIET	HIGHER PROTEIN DIET
Cold Turkey, Tomato Slices	Same
Tea, lemon wedge	Tea, plain

Dinner

Green Pepper Stuffed with Ground Beef	Same
Watercress	Same
Assorted Cheeses	None
Coffee, heavy cream	Coffee, black

Snack

Cold Turkey	Same

FOURTEENTH DAY

Breakfast

Salami and Eggs	Same
Coffee, heavy cream	Coffee, black

Lunch

Canned Salmon	Same
Spinach Leaf Salad, Dressing	Same
Iced Tea, lemon wedge	Same

Dinner

Broiled Flank Steak	Same
Kale	Same
Peach Halves (two, drain sugar)	Peach Half (one, drain sugar)
Coffee, heavy cream	Coffee, plain

Snack

Cold Flank Steak	Same

FIFTEENTH DAY

Breakfast

Orange Juice, 6 oz.	Orange, medium
Eggs any style, Bacon	Same
Coffee, heavy cream	Coffee, black

Lunch

Avocado with Turkey Salad	Turkey Salad
Diet Cola	Same

Dinner

Broiled Pork Chops	Same

HIGH PROTEIN DIET	HIGHER PROTEIN DIET
Spinach	Same
Diet Gelatin Dessert	Same
Coffee, heavy cream	Coffee, black

Snack

Cold Pork Chop	Same

SIXTEENTH DAY

Breakfast

Half Grapefruit	Same
Fried Eggs with Canadian Bacon	Same
Coffee, heavy cream	Coffee, black

Lunch

Roquefort Sliced Tomatoes (see recipes)	Same
Tea, lemon wedge	Tea, plain

Dinner

Indian Lobster (see recipes)	Same
Swiss Chard	Same
Camembert Dessert Mold (see recipes)	Selected Cheeses
Coffee, heavy cream	Coffee, black

Snack

Cheese	Hard Boiled Egg

SEVENTEENTH DAY

Breakfast

Small Breakfast Steak	Same
Coffee, heavy cream	Coffee, black

Lunch

Broiled Chicken Livers, Mushrooms	Same
Diet Soda	Same

Dinner

Flounder in Wine Sauce (see recipes)	Same
Braised Celery	Same
Radishes and Scallions	Same
½ Cantaloupe	¼ Cantaloupe
Coffee, heavy cream	Coffee, black

Snack

Hard Boiled Egg	Cheese

HIGH PROTEIN DIET	HIGHER PROTEIN DIET

EIGHTEENTH DAY

Breakfast

½ Cantaloupe	¼ Cantaloupe
Shirred Eggs	Same
Coffee, heavy cream	Coffee, black

Lunch

| Cauliflower au Gratin | Same |
| Diet Cola | Same |

Dinner

Roast Veal	Same
Mixed Salad, Dressing	Same
Coffee, heavy cream	Coffee, black

Snack

| Cold Veal | Same |

NINETEENTH DAY

Breakfast

| Mixed Grill (Bacon, Ham, Sausage) | Same |
| Coffee, heavy cream | Coffee, black |

Lunch

Cold Veal	Same
Light Salad	Same
Tea, lemon wedge	Tea, plain

Dinner

Broiled Chicken	Same
Boiled Creamed Onions	Boiled Onions
Berries, heavy cream	Berries, plain
Coffee, black	Same

Snack

| Cold Chicken | Same |

TWENTIETH DAY

Breakfast

Berries, plain	Same
Scrambled Eggs, Bacon	Same
Coffee, heavy cream	Coffee, black

HIGH PROTEIN DIET	HIGHER PROTEIN DIET
	Lunch
Shrimp and Egg Curry (see recipes)	Shrimp Salad
Diet Soda	Same
	Dinner
Lamb Chops	Same
Summer Squash	Same
Selected Cheeses	None
Coffee, heavy cream	Coffee, black
	Snack
Cold Chicken	Same

TWENTY-FIRST DAY

	Breakfast
Creamed Cod	Same
Coffee, black	Same
	Lunch
Reheated Lamb Chops	Same
Olives and Celery	Same
Tea, lemon wedge	Tea, plain
	Dinner
Pot Roast	Same
Turnips	Same
Half Grapefruit	Same
Coffee, heavy cream	Coffee, black
	Snack
Cold Pot Roast	Same

TWENTY-SECOND DAY

	Breakfast
Half Grapefruit	Same
Fried Eggs with Ham	Same
Coffee, heavy cream	Coffee, black
	Lunch
Beef Bouillon	Same
Cold Pot Roast	Same
Diet Cola .	Same

HIGH PROTEIN DIET	HIGHER PROTEIN DIET

Dinner

Flounder in Wine Sauce	Same
Broccoli à la Francaise (see recipes)	Steamed Broccoli
Diet Gelatin Dessert	Same
Coffee, heavy cream	Coffee, black

Snack

| Cheese | Leftover Meat or Fish |

TWENTY-THIRD DAY

Breakfast

V-8 Juice (6 oz.)	Half Grapefruit
Reheated Flounder	Same
Coffee, heavy cream	Coffee, black

Lunch

| Hamburger Steak, Watercress | Same |
| Tea, lemon wedge | Same |

Dinner

Boiled Tongue, Pickles	Same
Sauerkraut	Same
Selected Cheeses	None
Coffee, heavy cream	Coffee, black

Snack

| Cold Tongue | Same |

TWENTY-FOURTH DAY

Breakfast

| Small Breakfast Steak | Same |
| Coffee, heavy cream | Coffee, black |

Lunch

Cold Tongue	Same
Sauerkraut	Same
Diet Soda	Same

Dinner

Spiced Kebabs (see recipes)	Same
Mixed Green Salad	Same
Zabaglione	Same

Snack

| Apple | Same |

HIGH PROTEIN DIET	HIGHER PROTEIN DIET

TWENTY-FIFTH DAY

Breakfast

Tangerine Juice (6 oz.)	Tangerine
Soft Boiled Eggs, Link Sausage	Same
Coffee, heavy cream	Coffee, black

Lunch

Artichoke and Watercress Salad (see recipes)	Same
Cheese	Leftover Meat or Fish
Tea, lemon wedge	Tea, plain

Dinner

Roast Ham	Same
Spinach	Same
Radishes	Radish
Coffee, heavy cream	Coffee, black

Snack

Cold Ham	Same

TWENTY-SIXTH DAY

Breakfast

Poached Eggs, Bacon	Same
Coffee, heavy cream	Coffee, black

Lunch

Ham Mold (see recipes)	Same
Tea, lemon wedge	Tea, plain

Dinner

T-Bone Steak	Same
Broiled Mushrooms	Same
Watercress	Same
Pineapple Slice (drain syrup)	Same
Coffee, heavy cream	Coffee, black

Snack

Cold Ham	Same

TWENTY-SEVENTH DAY

Breakfast

Orange Juice (6 oz.)	Orange, medium
Scrambled Eggs, Portuguese Sausage	Same
Coffee, heavy cream	Coffee, black

HIGH PROTEIN DIET   ## HIGHER PROTEIN DIET

Lunch

Breakfast Steak, Watercress	Same
Tea, lemon wedge	Tea, plain

Dinner

Cream of Mushroom Soup	
Roast Squab or Guinea Hen	Same
Stewed Tomatoes	Same
Gelatin Dessert	Same
Coffee, heavy cream	Coffee, plain

Snack

Leftover Poultry	Same

TWENTY-EIGHTH DAY

Breakfast

Ham and Eggs, any style	Same
Coffee, heavy cream	Coffee, black

Lunch

Shrimp Salad	Same
Cheese	Leftover Meat or Fish
Diet Cola	Same

Dinner

Chicken Eggplant (see recipes)	Broiled Chicken
Spinach Leaf Salad	Spinach
Custard	Tangerine

Snack

Tangerine	Cold Chicken

TWENTY-NINTH DAY

Breakfast

Ham Steak	Same
Coffee, heavy cream	Coffee, black

Lunch

Chicken Bouillon	Same
Deviled Eggs	Same
Tea, lemon wedge	Tea, plain

Dinner

Pacific Veal (see recipes)	Veal Stew

HIGH PROTEIN DIET	HIGHER PROTEIN DIET
Chinese Cabbage	Same
Mixed Green Salad	Same
Apricots (three, syrup drained)	Apricots (two, syrup drained)

Snack

Deviled Egg	Same

THIRTIETH DAY

Breakfast

Sliced Veal, Natural Gravy	Same
Coffee, heavy cream	Coffee, black

Lunch

Beef Bouillon	Same
Selected Cheese	Leftover Meat or Fish
Diet Cola	Same

Dinner

Hamburger Steak	Same
Onions and Mushrooms	Same
Half Grapefruit	Same
Coffee, heavy cream	Coffee, black

Snack

Leftover Hamburger	Same

8

FAT DESTROYING RECIPES
FOR SUMPTUOUS DINING

Some couples grow old together. Stanley and Olivia grew fat together. Olivia was a great cook. Stanley appreciated her cooking. Olivia enjoyed it, too.

Olivia's family was Italian. Stanley's family was Jewish. So Olivia knew how to cook lasagna, matzoh balls, fettucini, potato latkes, spaghetti, etc. It did not matter which family was coming to dinner that night, or if it was just to be a twosome. She made the most wonderful clam sauce and "cholent," a slow-baked meat dish, which, to the uninformed, also contains two pounds of potatoes, one pound of lima beans, and a few other carbohydrate ingredients looking for a body to call their home.

Needless to say, Stanley and Olivia were blossoming. Neither one had ever considered that gourmet foods could also be non-fattening foods. Among traditional Jewish foods, there are appetizers such as chopped herring which consists of herring and onion, lemon, hard-boiled egg and vegetable oil; and there is gefilte fish, which is a combination of pike, whitefish and carp, onions, eggs, a little celery, a little carrot and salt and pepper.

There is even a dish for the very brave called "Pitcha," which consists of one calf's foot, one onion, one clove of garlic, one bay leaf, the juice of a small lemon, two tablespoons of white vinegar, and two sliced hard-boiled eggs.

Believe it or not, entrees such as corned beef and cabbage, Hungarian goulash, Russian goulash, sweetbreads, fried liver and onions, lamb stew, veal stew, meatballs with mushrooms, pot roast, Swiss steak,—all are high-protein, low-carbohydrate dishes.

For the Italian taste there are, of course, the great antipastos, clams in garlic sauce, shrimp scampi and all of the delicious veal dishes, sauteed with lemon and butter and with that fine garlic touch. There is veal parmigiana which does not have to be breaded but is covered with that delicious cheese and tomato topping. Boned chicken breasts, rolled with paper-thin slices of prosciutto, sautéed in butter and flavored with tarragon, is a meal fit for any king or dieter.

Thanks to fat destroying protein foods, Stanley and Olivia are slender now. They discovered what you can discover—that gourmet foods do not have to include heavy, thick, fattening starches, sugars, or those other villains that, taken by mouth, find a home in your waistline.

The Basic Recipe for Protein Diets

Take a fat destroying protein, add a sprinkle of exotic flavor, bake in warm love and serve with enthusiasm.

That's the basic recipe for thousands of taste-tempting dishes that make the High Protein Diet and even the Higher Protein Diet a gourmet way of life.

The scores of recipes in the pages ahead are only a soupcon of the possibilities that await you. They have been tested and tasted by myself and the wives and friends of my associates and clients. Many come from their files and therefore may have unknown original sources. We apologize to these sources if we have adapted them and they have lost some of their original savor in the translation, or if we have not adapted them and thus made them appear as our own.

I hereby give credit where credit is due—to some enterprising gourmet who has put together a high protein dish worthy of the hall of high protein fame.

How to Cook So As to Make Every Calorie Count
Toward Hunger-Preventing Nutrition

You can buy nutritious foods. Yet, when you serve them, they can be closer to empty calories.

Where have all the nutrients gone?

1. They have become oxidized in storage.
2. They have dissolved in the cooking water.
3. They have been burned up in the heat.

Slam these doors and you lock in the original nutrients. Or at least close them as much as is feasible.

You can't go marketing everyday, so your salad material will begin to wilt, unless you buy the crispest heads and store them in the coolest (bottom) part of your refrigerator.

You can't cook all your meals in the oven, but you can use less water when you cook on top of the stove.

You can't cook without heat, but you can use lower heat and you can begin to enjoy your meat closer to medium rare or rare, or even very rare.

If you are on the Highest Protein (Crash) Diet, it is best to limit fats, too. Low-fat cookery uses Teflon-type pans for frying. Broiling is preferred, so that the fat can drip away. Remember that one forkful of fatty food provides twice the caloric value of protein food without any increase in nutrition and probably a decrease.

"Go" Signs and "Stop" Signs in Gourmet Cooking
for the High Protein Diets

"Open two cans of potato soup." You are reading a favorite recipe of yours from the old, more fattening days. Of course, you go no further. Potatoes are carbohydrate foods. Next recipe.

Every recipe must be examined with a carbohydrate-conscious eye. If it calls for one tablespoon of flour per portion, you may be blowing your diet for the day. One tablespoon of flour for four to six portions is passable.

Other carbohydrate pitfalls are bread crumbs, sugar, cornstarch, nuts (except for just a sprinkling), and dried fruits (like raisins).

Sometimes, special casseroles call for beans or apples or other high starch vegetables and fruits. These are to be avoided, or else portions are to be cut in half. Of course, where one portion of vegetable or fruit is permitted and a meat, fish, or, poultry casserole contains fruit or vegetable, this counts for the portion of fruit or vegetable.

Cooking with wine

Dry wines may be used in cooking but not sweet wines. This is true even for the standard High Protein Diet where alcoholic beverages are not permitted, because cooking causes the alcohol to vaporize off.

If in doubt, use the table at the center of this book to guide you. The right-hand column tells you the carbohydrate calories, or carbo-cals, in typical portions of various foods. If you want to put your favorite recipe through the test, total the carbo-cals and divide the number of persons it serves.

Carbo-Cal Allotment

Maximum total daily allotment of carbo-cals is as follows:

	High Protein Diet	Higher Protein Diet	Highest Protein Diet
Maximum carbo-cals allowed daily	200	100	trace

If your recipe uses up your daily allowance of carbo-cals, that means no portion of fruit, no portion of vegetable and no salad that day.

Not included in these recipes are the simple dishes that require no "special" preparation.

You don't need a recipe to roast beef, or broil chops, or boil eggs, or melt cheese, or steam vegetables, or fry bacon.

You really don't need any recipes, as you can create in the kitchen as well as anyone else.

But, at least, these may inspire you.
Happy dining.

Recipes That Use Fat Destroying Foods

SOUP

Blender Soup

1/2 cup sliced celery	1 carrot
1 cup sliced cucumber	1 tablespoon chopped onion
1/2 green pepper, cut up	2 cups tomato juice
watercress or parsley	salt and pepper to taste

Put the vegetables slowly into the blender. Do not put too much in at one time, or the blender will not chop them fine enough. When all the vegetables have become liquified, slowly add the tomato juice and salt and pepper. Blend all together thoroughly. Garnish with chives.

Hot Protein Broth

Blend 2 eggs until foamy. Heat 1 cup regular strength chicken or beef broth to boiling; quickly blend in eggs. Pour into a mug; top with a little shredded Parmesan cheese, freshly grated pepper. Makes 1 serving

Hot Milk Broth

Whirl 1 or 2 eggs until foamy in a covered blender jar. Heat to scalding, stirring, 1 cup milk, 1/2 teaspoon butter and 1 chicken or beef bouillon cube, crumbled. Pour hot liquid into blending eggs. Serve in a large mug and sprinkle lightly with pepper and shredded Parmesan cheese. Makes 1 serving.

POULTRY

Chicken Curry

1 tablespoon butter or fat	1/2 teaspoon salt

1 tablespoon chopped onion   1/8 teaspoon pepper
1 tablespoon flour   2 cups stock or chicken bouillon
1 teaspoon curry powder   1 1/2 cups cooked chicken,
                                       chopped

Melt fat, add onion and cook to a light brown. Add flour, curry powder, salt and pepper and mix well. Add stock slowly and bring to boiling point, stirring constantly, until mixture is smooth and slightly thickened. Add chicken and allow to heat thoroughly. Garnish with parsley and serve with chutney. Serves 2.

Chicken Eggplant Tokyo

Cut up chicken fryer into serving pieces. Cut one large eggplant into 6 rounds; then halve. Mix together 1 cup soy sauce; 1/4 teaspoon powdered ginger; 1 clove of garlic, chopped; and a dash of cayenne. Stir in 1/2 cup chopped green onion. Marinate chicken and eggplant for 1/2 hour. Broil or barbecue for 30-45 minutes, basting and turning occasionally. Serves 4 to 6.

Chicken Salad Super

1 1/2 cups mayonnaise   2 tablespoons soy sauce
1/4 cup lemon juice   2 cups diced celery
6 cups cooked, diced   ½ cup slivered almonds
   turkey or chicken   1 can chicken broth

To the broth, add 1 medium onion, 2 celery tops, finely cut, 2 bay leaves, dash of pepper. For salad, mix mayonnaise, lemon juice and soy sauce. Toss lightly with cubed chicken or turkey, celery and almonds. Chill. Serve with sliced melon.

Chicken with Olives and Lemons

3 to 3 1/2 pound chicken   7 ounces of black olives
1 onion, finely chopped   3 preserved lemons (to preserve,
Bunch of parsley and   sprinkle lemon slices
   coriander, finely chopped   heavily with salt and
1/4 teaspoon saffron (optional)   refrigerate for 3 days
1/2 teaspoon black pepper   before using)
1/2 cup olive oil

In heavy pot, put onion, garlic, coriander and parsley, saffron and pepper, lay trussed chicken on top, half cover with water and add salt to taste. Cover and bring to a boil. Add olive oil, turn chicken occasionally. When flesh is soft, about 40 minutes, remove chicken and reduce sauce by simmering uncovered until water has completely evaporated. Replace chicken, simmer for a few minutes, garnish with olives and sliced lemons, pour sauce over and serve. Serves 3.

Chicken Palau

Boil chicken fryer in a pot half filled with water. Peel skin off and chop boiled meat into tiny pieces. Put chicken meats on tray. Add salt, pepper, lemon, grated coconut, red pepper and finely chopped onions. Mix and serve.

MEAT

"Bisteak"

Slice beef into 2" pieces. Put salad oil into pot. Saute onions in pot till they are brown. Mix salt, black pepper, vinegar, and soy sauce with meat. Add this mixture to pot containing salad oil and cook until there is no more meat juice.

Flank Steak with Olives

1 pound flank steak, cut in thin strips	1/2 teaspoon salt dash of pepper
1 tablespoon salad oil	1 tablespoon vinegar
1/2 large onion, chopped	5 ounces tomato paste
1 medium green pepper, cut in thin strips	1/4 cup halved pimento-stuffed olives
1 clove garlic, minced	

Brown meat on both sides in oil in skillet. Drain off the drippings. Mix remaining ingredients, except olives, with meat. Cover and cook over low heat 1 hour or until meat is tender. Now add olives and heat 5 minutes. Makes 2 servings.

Hekka

Slice 2 pounds beef or chicken or pork into very thin slices, about 2 inches long. Slice diagonally 1 bunch green onions and enough watercress to make 1 cup. Slice 1 pound mushrooms. Slice bamboo shoots or bean sprouts to make 1/2 cup. Heat 1 cup soy sauce. Add onions, mushrooms, bamboo shoots, and watercress. Finally, stir in meat and cook for a few minutes. Serves 4.

Israeli Curried Beef

Combine in saucepan 1/2 can tomato soup, 1 cup dry sherry, and 1 cup water. Add 1 bay leaf, 1/4 teaspoon curry powder, and a dash of mace, cumin, marjoram, and red pepper. Add 1 teaspoon salt and 1 large clove garlic, minced. Simmer for 30 minutes.

Brown 1 1/2 pounds bite-size beef chuck in 2 tablespoons peanut oil; add sauce and simmer until tender, about 2 hours. Stir in 2 cups onion slices, 4 carrots, quartered lengthwise, and 1 cup sliced celery. Simmer for 15 minutes; add 1 cup watercress or 1/2 cup parsley, chopped, and continue cooking 5 minutes. Serves 4 to 6.

Liver and Bacon with Cabbage

1 pound beef or calf liver	2 tablespoons salad oil
4 tablespoons soy sauce	medium head shredded cabbage
8 slices bacon	1 large onion, sliced
2 tablespoons dry wine	

Cut liver into bite-sized pieces; place in a bowl with 3 tablespoons of the soy sauce, let stand 1/4 hour. Drain. Pierce one end of a bacon strip with a small skewer. Add on a piece of liver. Thread bacon over and under 2 or 3 more pieces of liver to the other end of the bacon slice. Broil skewers on the rack of a broiler pan, about 4 inches from heat, turning until bacon is crisp. Heat oil in a wok, add cabbage and onion, cover, and cook over medium heat, stirring often, until cabbage is tender, about 9 minutes. Stir in the remaining soy sauce and wine; top with skewers. Serves 4.

Pacific Veal

For each serving, cut 12-inch square of aluminum foil. Place 3 cubes veal, 3 chunks pineapple, 1 tablespoon chopped green pepper, 1 chopped tomato, sprinkle with chopped peanuts, and dash of red pepper or ginger. Seal packages. Bake in medium oven (350 degrees) for about 1 1/2 hours.

Spiced Kebabs

1 pound ground round steak
1 cup hot water
2 teaspoons salt
1 stick cinnamon, 2" long
1 whole ginger, 1 1/2" long
1 teaspoon instant minced
  onion
1 teaspoon water
1/4 teaspoon ground red
  pepper
1/4 teaspoon ground
  cardamom seed

1/4 teaspoon garlic powder
1/2 teaspoon finely crumbled
  mint flakes
2/3 cup water
1 tablespoon instant
  minced onion
1 tablespoon water
1 egg
1 tablespoon milk
1 teaspoon ground black pepper

Cook together, uncovered, in a saucepan, meat, 1 cup hot water, salt, cinnamon and ginger 35 minutes or until all water has evaporated and the meat is very dry. Put meat in a strainer and press out all the excess fat. Soften instant minced onion in the 1 teaspoon water and add to the meat. Mix and put through a food chopper using the finest blade. Repeat to grind meat very fine. Add spices. Mix well. Add the 2/3 cup water. Stir and cook over medium heat, about 5 minutes until meat holds together when squeezed. Cool enough to handle (about 5 minutes). Shape 1 rounded tablespoon meat into a 2-inch patty. Soften remaining 1 tablespoon instant minced onion in the 1 tablespoon water. Place ¼ teaspoon in center of each patty. Pull meat over the onion until it is no longer visible. Beat together egg and milk into which dip meat balls. Brown in deep fat preheated to 375 F. Drain on paper towels. Yield: 10 kebabs, each 2" in diameter.

FISH

Aioli

On a tray, place each of the following foods separately: cold oven-steamed fish (directions below); 4 hard-cooked, cold eggs; 1 bunch trimmed radishes; 2 sliced green peppers; sliced tomatoes; green onions, arranging attractively. Sprinkle the fish with paprika. Accompany with aioli sauce (directions follow). Makes 4 servings.

Oven-steamed fish. Place 1 pound boneless fish fillets in a pan. Add 2 tablespoons vinegar and sprinkle lightly with salt. Cover and bake fish

in a 400° oven, 12 to 14 minutes. Chill thoroughly in a baking pan.
Aioli sauce. Blend 1 cup mayonnaise with 2 teaspoons mustard and 1
teaspoon minced garlic. Cover and chill several hours.

✓ Broiled Yellow Perch

2 pounds yellow perch fillets
 or other fish fillets,
 fresh or frozen
1/4 cup butter or margarine,
 melted
2 tablespoons lemon juice

2 tablespoons chopped parsley
1/2 teaspoon salt
1/8 teaspoon pepper
Paprika
Lemon wedges

Skin thawed fillets and place on a greased broil and serve platter,
16 x 10 inches. Combine remaining ingredients except paprika and
lemon wedges. Pour over fillets and let stand for 30 minutes. Broil
about 4 inches from source of heat for 8 to 10 minutes or until fish
flakes easily when tested with a fork. Sprinkle with paprika. Serve with
lemon wedges. Serves 6.

Curried Cod

2 pounds cod fillets or
 other fish fillets,
 fresh or frozen
1 cup thinly sliced celery
1 cup thinly sliced onion
3/4 cup skim milk

1 tablespoon melted fat
 or oil
1 teaspoon curry powder
1 teaspoon salt
Dash pepper
Paprika

Skin thawed fillets and place in a single layer in a greased baking dish,
12 x 8 x 2 inches. Cook the celery and onion in fat for 5 minutes. Stir
in seasonings and milk. Spread over fish. Bake in a moderate oven, 350°
F., for 25 to 30 minutes or until fish flakes easily when tested with a
fork. Sprinkle with paprika. Serves 6.

Fillet of Sole Hawaii

4 fillets of sole or other
 fish
salt and pepper
3 tablespoons salad oil

2 tablespoons lemon or
 lime juice
1 large avocado
1/4 cup yogurt

Season fillets with salt and pepper; sprinkle with 1 tablespoon lemon juice and let stand 10 minutes. Halve and seed avocado. Cut fruit into cubes.

Heat oil in skillet. Brown fillets. Add yogurt and half of avocado cubes; heat minute or two.

Remove fillets to serving dish; top with remainder of avocado cubes and lemon juice. Pour mixture over the top. Sprinkle with rest of lemon juice. Serves 4.

Flounder in Wine Sauce

2 pounds flounder fillets or
    other fish fillets,
    fresh or frozen
1 1/2 teaspoons salt
Dash pepper
3 tomatoes, sliced
Chopped parsley

1 tablespoon flour
2 tablespoons butter or
    margarine, melted
1/2 cup milk
1/3 cup dry white wine
1/2 teaspoon crushed basil

Skin thawed fillets. Sprinkle fillets on both sides with salt and pepper. Place fillets in a single layer in a greased baking dish, 12 x 8 x 2 inches. Arrange tomatoes over top of fillets. Sprinkle with salt and pepper. Blend flour into butter. Add milk gradually and cook until thick and smooth, stirring constantly. Remove from heat and stir in wine and basil. Pour sauce over top of tomatoes. Bake in a moderate oven, 350°F., for 25 to 30 minutes or until fish flakes easily when tested with a fork. Sprinkle with parsley. Serves 6.

Halibut Mornay

Place 4 halibut steaks (3 lbs.), cut about 3/4 inch thick, in a shallow, buttered baking dish. Sprinkle lightly with salt and pepper. In a bowl, mix together 3/4 cup yogurt, 1/4 teaspoon minced garlic, and 1 1/2 tablespoons chopped chives. Spread mixture over fish; sprinkle about 1/3 cup grated Parmesan cheese over yogurt. Sprinkle 1 teaspoon paprika over the surface. Bake uncovered in a hot oven for about 20 minutes or until fish flakes with a fork. Garnish with parsley and lemon wedges. Makes 4 large servings.

Hearty Halibut

2 pounds halibut steaks or
    other fish steaks,
    fresh or frozen

1/4 cup chopped parsley
3 tablespoons chopped pimento
1/2 cup dry white wine

2/3 cup thinly sliced onion
1 1/2 cups chopped fresh
    mushrooms
1/3 cup chopped tomato
1/4 cup chopped green pepper

2 tablespoons lemon juice
1 teaspoon salt
1/4 teaspoon dill weed
1/8 teaspoon pepper
Lemon wedges

Thaw steaks if frozen. Cut into serving-size portions. Arrange onion in bottom of a greased baking dish, 12 x 8 x 2 inches. Place fish on top of onion. Combine remaining vegetables and spread over top of fish. Combine wine, lemon juice, and seasonings. Pour over vegetables. Bake in a moderate oven, 350° F., for 25 to 30 minutes or until fish flakes easily when tested with a fork. Serve with lemon wedges. Serves 6.

Key Lime Mullet

2 pounds mullet fillets or
    other fish fillets,
    fresh or frozen
1 teaspoon salt
dash pepper

1/4 cup lime juice
3 tablespoons butter or
    margarine, melted
Paprika
Lime wedges

Skin thawed fillets and cut into serving-size portions. Place fish in a single layer in a shallow baking dish. Sprinkle with salt and pepper. Pour lime juice over fish and let stand for 30 minutes, turning once. Remove fish, reserving juice. Place fish on a well-greased broiler pan. Combine butter and juice. Brush fish with butter mixture and sprinkle with paprika. Broil about 4 inches from source of heat for 8 to 10 minutes or until fish flakes easily when tested with a fork. Serve with lime wedges. Serves 6.

Lisbon Fish Stew

4 tablespoons olive oil
2/3 cup onion, chopped
1 clove garlic, minced
1 medium-sized green pepper,
    chopped
1 medium-sized carrot, chopped
2 medium-sized tomatoes, cut up

1/2 teaspoon each salt,
    paprika, and thyme
1 bay leaf
1 1/2 pounds fish fillet
1 pound medium-sized shrimp,
    shelled and deveined
4 tablespoons minced parsley

1 cup regular-strength
  beef broth
1/2 cup dry white wine

2 green onions, chopped fine
1 package frozen peas

In a large kettle, heat olive oil, add the onion and garlic and brown. Add the green pepper, carrot, tomatoes, broth, wine, and seasonings. Bring mixture to a boil, reduce heat and simmer for 1/4 hour. Cut the fish into 1-inch cubes and add to the pan; simmer for 2 minutes. Add the shrimp and cook until they turn firm and pink, about 3 minutes. Add peas. Serve in a deep serving bowl. Sprinkle with parsley. Makes 6 servings.

Salmon Paysanne

2 pounds salmon steaks or
  other fish steaks,
  fresh or frozen
1/2 teaspoon salt
1/4 teaspoon white pepper
1/2 cup sliced green onions

1 can (4 ounces) sliced
  mushrooms, drained
1/4 cup catsup
2 tablespoons butter or
  margarine, melted
1/2 teaspoon liquid smoke

Thaw frozen steaks. Cut into serving-size portions. Place in a greased baking dish, 12 x 8 x 2 inches. Sprinkle with salt and pepper. Combine remaining ingredients and spread over top of fish. Bake in a moderate oven, 350° F., for 25 to 30 minutes or until fish flakes easily when tested with a fork. Serves 6.

Savory Baked Haddock

2 pounds haddock fillets or
  other fish fillets,
  fresh or frozen
2 teaspoons lemon juice
Dash pepper

6 slices bacon, chopped
1/2 cup soft bread crumbs
2 tablespoons chopped parsley
3/4 cup thinly sliced onion
2 tablespoons bacon fat

Skin thawed fillets and place in a single layer in a greased baking dish, 12 x 8 x 2 inches. Sprinkle with lemon juice and pepper. Fry bacon until crisp. Remove bacon from fat. Add to bread crumbs and parsley. Cook onion in bacon fat until tender. Spread onion over fish. Sprinkle crumb mixture over top of onion. Bake in a moderate oven, 350° F., for 25 to 30 minutes or until fish flakes easily when tested with a fork. Serves 6.

Spicy Snapper

2 pounds snapper fillets or
   other fish fillets,
   fresh or frozen
2/3 cup tomato juice
3 tablespoons vinegar

2 tablespoons salad oil
1 envelope (5/8 ounce) old-
   fashioned French dressing
   mix

Skin thawed fillets and cut into serving-size portions. Place fish in a single layer in a shallow baking dish. Combine remaining ingredients and mix thoroughly. Pour sauce over fish and let stand for 30 minutes, turning once. Remove fish, reserving sauce for basting. Place fish on a well-greased broiler pan. Broil about 4 inches from source of heat for 4 to 5 minutes. Turn carefully and brush with sauce. Broil 4 to 5 minutes longer or until fish flakes easily when tested with a fork. Serves 6.

SEA FOOD

Hot Lobster Salad

Sauté 1 tablespoon each finely chopped celery and onion; add 1/4 cup mayonnaise seasoned to taste with Worcestershire and Tabasco. Heat. Add 1/2 cup diced lobster meat. Heat thoroughly. Serve on chilled lettuce.

Indian Lobster

3-pound lobster, parboiled
8 tablespoons oil
1/2 teaspoon salt
1 tablespoon chopped fresh
   ginger or 1/4 teaspoon
   powdered ginger
1 1/2 quarts buttermilk

5 onions, sliced
5 cardamom seeds
1/4 teaspoon saffron
1 1/2 tablespoons coriander
2 teaspoons black pepper
3 tablespoons lemon juice

Extract lobster meat. Heat 3 tablespoons oil and cook the lobster quickly. Pound the salt with the ginger and 2 tablespoons water. Add the buttermilk. Strain over the lobster. Cover and simmer for 15 minutes. Remove lobster and reserve sauce.

Brown the onions in rest of oil with the cardamom seeds. Cover, turn the heat high and give the pan a good shake. Add the saffron, coriander, black pepper and 2 tablespoons lemon juice. Cover, raise heat high and again shake well. Meanwhile, simmer the buttermilk sauce with 1 tablespoon lemon juice. Reduce liquid by half, add the lobster.

Indian Shrimp

1 pound raw American-type shrimp	12 black peppercorns
salad oil	1 1/2 teaspoons salt
1/2 cup boiling water	1/2 teaspoon ground cumin seed
1 teaspoon salt	1 teaspoon ground turmeric
1 teaspoon ground coriander	2 teaspoons fresh lemon or
1/2 teaspoon instant minced onion	lime juice
	8 wedges fresh lemon or lime

Peel and devein raw shrimp. Set aside. Place in a saucepan with boiling water, the 1 teaspoon salt, 1/2 teaspoon of the coriander, instant minced onion and black peppercorns. Bring to boiling point. Add peeled shrimp and cook 2 minutes or until shrimp begin to turn pink. Remove from heat and drain off water. Add oil, salt, remaining spices and lemon or lime juice. Mix well. Stir in shrimp. Turn into a shallow pan. Spread over surface. Broil 5 minutes or until shrimp are pink and slightly browned around the edges. Serve with a wedge of fresh lime or lemon. Yield: 8 servings, 5 shrimp for each.

Shrimp and Egg Curry

1 medium onion, chopped	1 tablespoon flour
1 garlic clove, minced	1 cup consommé
2 tablespoons salad oil	1 teaspoon salt
1/2 cup diced celery	1/4 teaspoon pepper
1 large green apple, peeled and diced	2 cups cleaned cooked or canned shrimp
1/2 teaspoon paprika	4 hard-cooked eggs, sliced
1 tablespoon curry powder	

Saute onion and garlic in salad oil until soft and yellow. Add celery and apple. Mix paprika, curry powder and flour and add to mixture; mix well. Add consommé gradually, stirring constantly until thickened. Add salt and pepper. Let simmer 30 minutes. Add shrimp and hard cooked eggs. Simmer 15 minutes longer. Serve with the following accompaniments: grated coconut, chutney, crystallized ginger, salted almonds and pickled onions. Approximate yield: 6 portions.

VEGETABLES

Broccoli à la Francaise

3/4 pound broccoli
2 slices bacon, fried crisp
    and crumbled
pinch of salt, pepper,
    nutmeg, ginger

2 eggs
3/4 cup light cream
2 tablespoons freshly shredded
    Parmesan cheese

Trim tough ends from broccoli. Cut off flowerets and reserve; slice stems crosswise 1/3 inch thick.
Drop broccoli stems into boiling water and cook 5 minutes, then add flowerets and boil until just tender. Drain and place into a shallow baking dish; sprinkle with the bacon. Combine seasonings and eggs, beaten lightly with a fork. Stir in cream and Parmesan and pour over broccoli.
Set baking dish inside a pan of hot water. Bake in a 350 degrees oven for 1/2 hour. Serve at once. Makes about 3 servings.

✓ Eggplant Italienne

1 large eggplant
2 medium onions, sliced
2 medium tomatoes, sliced
olive oil

3/4 cup sharp cheese,
    shredded
salt, pepper, paprika

Slice the eggplant into 1/2-inch pieces. Place by layers in a casserole. Season and add a little of the cheese. Continue layering. Sprinkle with oil and paprika, cover and bake 45 minutes in a moderate oven. Uncover and bake until cheese starts to brown. Serves 4.

Japanese Cauliflower

Steam a small cauliflower on rack for 20 minutes in 1/2 cup water with 1 1/2 teaspoons vinegar.
Drain and cool; break into florets. Serve with sauce. Makes 6.

Sauce: Mix 3 tablespoons mayonnaise with 3 tablespoons yogurt; sprinkle with vinegar, lime juice, pepper, and salt.

Marinated Mushroom Platter

1 1/2 pounds mushrooms	3/4 teaspoon tarragon,
1/2 pound Gruyère cheese	crumbled
2 cups celery, sliced fine	parsley
1/4 cup vinegar	dash of powdered ginger
1/2 cup salad oil	squeeze of garlic juice

Wash mushrooms; pat dry. Cut into thin slices; place in a bowl. Sliver cheese, place in another bowl with celery.

In a small jar or bowl combine the lemon juice, oil, tarragon, ginger, garlic juice. Shake to blend. Pour half the dressing over the mushrooms and the remainder over the cheese and celery; mix. Cover each and refrigerate overnight, stirring gently several times.

Carefully arrange mushrooms and cheese and celery on a shallow platter. Garnish with parsley. Drizzle with remaining marinade. Makes about 10 servings.

Roquefort Sliced Tomatoes

2 firm, ripe tomatoes	1/4 cup crumbled Roquefort
salad greens	or Blue cheese
1/2 Bermuda onion	1/2 cup salad oil
1/4 cup minced parsley	2 tablespoons lemon juice
1/2 teaspoon salt	

Thinly slice tomatoes, place on greens arranged on a large plate. Slice onion very thinly and place a slice on each tomato. Sprinkle with parsley. Blend together the Roquefort cheese, salad oil, lemon juice, and salt. Pour dressing over the tomatoes and chill at least 20 minutes before serving. Serves 3.

Spicy Cheese Tomatoes

4 medium-sized firm tomatoes	2 tablespoons chopped green
1/2 pint (1 cup) sour cream	onion
salt and pepper to taste	1 tablespoon green chiles
1 cup (about 1/4 pound) shredded	
Cheddar cheese	

Thickly slice tomatoes. Remove some of the seeds. Arrange the tomatoes, with cut sides up, on the rack of a broiler pan. Combine the sour cream with salt, pepper, green onion, and chiles; stir well. Spoon mixture over the tomatoes and then sprinkle with cheese.

Broil until the cheese is bubbly about 4 minutes. The tomatoes will be just warm. Makes 8 servings.

Vegetable Casserole

1 package frozen artichoke hearts	1/4 cup milk
	garlic, salt and pepper
1 package frozen chopped spinach or broccoli	2 tomatoes, quartered
	1/2 cup mayonnaise
1/4 pound fresh mushrooms	1/2 cup plain yogurt
4 tablespoons butter	2 tablespoons lemon juice

Place the artichoke hearts in a casserole. Cook broccoli and drain. Slice the mushrooms, reserving a few slices for garnishing and sauté them in butter.

Add the milk, seasonings, broccoli, mushrooms, tomatoes, and pour over the artichokes in the casserole. Stir together the yogurt and mayonnaise and heat and add the lemon juice. Pour over the vegetables. Heat for 20 minutes at 350 degrees. Serves 4.

SALADS

Apple Salad

1 small avocado, diced	1/2 cup sharp cheddar cheese cubes
1/2 cup grapefruit sections	1 can tuna
1 cup diced unpeeled red apples	greens

Combine first four ingredients. Break tuna into pieces. Toss to mix. Arrange on crisp greens. Just before serving, toss again, with salad dressing. Makes 3 servings.

Artichokes and Watercress Salad

Drain 1 package frozen artichoke hearts. Mix with 1 tablespoon cider vinegar, 2 tablespoons olive oil, and 1 minced garlic clove, cover and let stand at room temperature for several hours. Wash 1 1/2 cups watercress leaves and drain. Sprinkle with the marinade and serve at once. Makes 3 servings.

Astoria Salad

4 cups diced apples   3/4 cup mayonnaise
2 cups celery, finely cut   chopped walnuts

In a bowl lightly mix the apples, celery and a sprinkling of walnuts. Add mayonnaise and mix gently but thoroughly. Serve on lettuce leaves.

Celery Salad

Slice 1 bunch celery into 1-inch chunks. Wash and scald for 2 minutes in 1 quart water. Remove and plunge into ice water for a minute. Drain; mix with 1 tablespoon soy sauce, 1 teaspoon sesame oil, 1 teaspoon sugar, and salt to taste. Chill. Serves 4.

Ham Mold

2 envelopes unflavored gelatin   1/2 cup mayonnaise
1 1/2 cups tomato juice   2 tablespoons pickle relish
1 tablespoon wine vinegar   2 cups finely chopped,
1/4 teaspoon paprika   cooked ham
1 tablespoon minced onion   1/2 cup finely diced Gruyere cheese
1 teaspoon mustard   1/2 cup finely diced green pepper

Sprinkle the gelatin over tomato juice in a pan; allow to soften for about 5 minutes, then heat and stir until the gelatin is completely dissolved. Remove from heat and stir in the vinegar, paprika, onion, and mustard until well blended. Cool.
Stir in the mayonnaise and relish into cooled gelatin until smooth. Add the ham, cheese, and green pepper. Pour into a 1-quart salad mold and chill until firm. To unmold, immerse mold in hottest tap water for 5 seconds; cover with serving plate and invert. Makes 4 servings.

Mushroom Bacon Salad

Raw mushrooms, thinly sliced and marinated, are the base of this salad.

1 pound medium-sized fresh
  mushrooms
3 green onions (including part
  of the green tops), thinly
  sliced (about 1/4 cup)
2/3 cup olive oil or salad oil
4 tablespoons lemon juice

1 teaspoon A-1 Sauce
1/2 teaspoon salt
1/8 teaspoon pepper
1/8 teaspoon dry ginger
12 thin slices bacon
1/2 pound raw spinach

Wash and dry the mushrooms. Cut into thin slices. In a blender or jar, combine the green onions, oil, lemon juice, A-1 sauce, salt, pepper, and ginger. Blend well, then pour over the mushrooms. Mix, cover and refrigerate for at least 4 hours or overnight; stirring several times.
Cook the bacon until crisp; drain. To serve, spoon the mushrooms and onions and washed spinach. Top with crumbled bacon. Drizzle with remaining marinade. Makes 6 to 8 servings.

Pacific Cucumber Salad

Slice cucumber and wash with salt. Rinse and place in bowl. Add vinegar, soy sauce, a little salad oil, black pepper and chopped red ginger, mix and serve.

Recycled Turkey Salad

1 package frozen broccoli
6 ounces Swiss cheese, cut
  in thin slices

small head butter lettuce
about 3/4 pound cooked turkey
  or chicken, thinly sliced

Cook and chill broccoli. Shortly before serving, arrange the lettuce, broccoli, cheese, and turkey on a serving tray. Serve with your favorite dressing. Serves 6.

Spinach and Pine Nut Salad

Spread 1/3 cup pine nuts in a large shallow pan. Bake in moderate oven for 5 minutes, stirring until golden. Cool, blend with 3 1/2 tablespoons olive oil, 1 1/2 tablespoons cider vinegar, sprinkle of ground nutmeg, 1/4 teaspoon grated lemon peel, 1/4 teaspoon tarragon. Let stand at room temperature 1/2 hour or longer. Wash and drain leaves from 3/4 pounds spinach. Tear into bite-size. Stir dressing to blend, in salad bowl toss altogether and serve. Makes 4 servings.

SUPPER OR APPETIZERS

Guacamole

1 avocado
1/4 cup mayonnaise
1/4 teaspoon salt
1/4 teaspoon chili powder
garlic clove
dash Tabasco

1 tablespoon lime juice
1/2 medium tomato, chopped
1/4 cup each: sliced green
  onion, chopped celery,
  green pepper

In blender place avocado, mayonnaise, seasonings and lime juice. Blend and add rest of ingredients; chill thoroughly. Put into avocado shell and garnish with crisp greens. Makes about 2 to 3 servings.

Thai Tuna

1 drained can tuna
1 small lime juice *plus*
2 tablespoons lemon juice *or*
3 tablespoons lemon juice

1/4 cup finely sliced celery
1/4 cup finely sliced green
  pepper or green onions
sprinkle of hot pepper

Mix all together on platter, arrange washed lettuce leaves (Bibb or head lettuce). To serve, fill leaves with tuna mixture. Top with chopped peanuts.

Vegetable Relish Dip

3/4 cup shredded cabbage
3/4 shredded carrot
3/4 cup chopped beet top
2 tablespoons chopped onion
2 teaspoons mustard

2 teaspoons vinegar
2 tablespoons mayonnaise
1 cup sour cream
salt and pepper

Combine the cabbage, carrot, greens and onion. Blend in the mustard, vinegar, and mayonnaise. Season to taste. Add sour cream, cover and chill. Garnish with chives. About 2 1/2 cups. Serve on cucumber slices.

Fondue Recipe

Make your favorite fondue recipe and instead of bread, use raw vegetables such as string beans, carrots, cauliflower, mushrooms, green pepper or celery. Wash and cut into bite-sized slices.

EGGS

Eggs Curry

2 onions	2 tablespoons yogurt
1 tablespoon curry powder	1 tablespoon salad oil
1/2 pint vegetable stock	8 hard-boiled eggs

Fry thinly sliced onions in oil until golden colored. Sprinkle with curry powder and blend. Add stock a little at a time, stirring to keep smooth. Cook for 15 minutes. Then add yogurt a little at a time, stirring constantly. Slice hard-boiled eggs and heat in the sauce until hot. Serve ·at once. Serves 4 to 5.

Eggs En Gelée

3 thin slices of ham cut into oval shapes	1 envelope, gelatin
6 tarragon leaves or scallions	watercress, parsley or cherry tomatoes for garnish
3 poached eggs, trimmed	(optional)

Make aspic per instructions on gelatin envelope. Use chilled, but still liquid.

Spoon a thin layer of aspic into cups used as molds. Place 2 tarragon leaves in each.

Place one poached egg and an oval of ham in each mold. Fill the mold with liquid aspic. Chill.

Unmold, dip and place on serving dish. Garnish with watercress, parsley and cherry tomatoes. Yield: 6 servings.

Note: If tarragon leaves are not available, cut the green part of scallions into leaflike decorations and use instead.

Eggs in Hot Sauce

5 fresh tomatoes, peeled	3 tablespoons oil
1/4 cup parsley, chopped	salt to taste
2 cloves garlic, minced	2 eggs per person
1/2 teaspoon black pepper	

Heat oil slightly on low flame, add rest of ingredients except eggs, mixing well. Simmer for about 5 minutes. Break eggs into sauce (do not stir), poach until done (about 3 minutes), remove and serve with some of the sauce in which they were cooked.

DESSERTS

Camembert Dessert Mold

1 envelope unflavored gelatin	1/8 teaspoon dry ginger
1/4 cup cold water	small bunch of grapes
8 ounces ripe Camembert at	wedges of melons, apples, etc.
room temperature	1 cup sour cream

Sprinkle the gelatin over the water; set aside. Cut off the rind from the Camembert. With wooden spoon, beat the Camembert until smooth; add the sour cream and ginger until well blended. Heat and stir the gelatin, until dissolved. Add to the cheese mixture and blend well. Pour into mold (3 cup size), cover and chill until firm. Unmold and garnish with the fruit. To serve, scoop small portions of the cream onto wedges of fruit to accompany with grapes. Makes about 12 servings.

Coffee Bavarian Cream

1 tablespoon plain gelatin	1/3 cup milk
2/3 cup strong black coffee	1 cup whipping cream
2 eggs, separated	1/2 teaspoon vanilla
1/3 cup sugar	

Sprinkle gelatin on top of cold coffee. Over low heat, beat egg yolks and add half of the sugar. Pour milk in gradually, stirring until mixture begins to thicken. Stir in gelatin-coffee mixture until dissolved and add vanilla, when removed from heat. Chill until slightly set. Now beat egg whites, gradually adding remaining sugar until stiff. Whip cream and fold egg whites and cream into gelatin mixture. Rinse out mold with cold water, fill and chill until firm. Serves 4.

Melon Melé

Choose an assortment of melons to make 2 quarts of balls (such as cantaloupe, watermelon, honeydew, Crenshaw or Persian). Use a melon ball cutter; or cut into bite-sized cubes. Combine in a bowl; cover and chill. To serve, pile melon balls in a shallow serving dish. Garnish top with mint sprig. Makes 6 servings.

Poached Pears

6 whole pears   1 piece lime rind
1 cup water   cinammon stick
1/3 cup dry red wine   mace

Mix wine and water, add rind and cinammon stick, and gently poach pears, until soft. If desired sweeten juice. Serve hot or chilled. Serves 6.

Zabaglione

2 egg yolks   2 tablespoon dry red wine
1 scant tablespoon honey

Place in saucepan, beat constantly to thicken over low heat. Spoon into wine glasses and serve warm. (Quantities shown are per serving.)

9

THE MAGIC METABOLIZING SANDWICH DIET
TO LOSE WEIGHT

Earlier, for those who cannot tolerate a high protein diet, I promised two highly effective diets.

In this chapter, I give you the Sandwich Diet. In the next chapter, the Rice Diet. Consult your physician as to their appropriateness for you.

Both of these diets are high in carbohydrates. Therefore, they must also be high in self-control and willpower on your part for them to succeed for you.

The higher the carbohydrates in a diet, the lower the calorie intake necessary for you to lose weight. So these are not permissive diets.

Both of these diets contain about 400 carbo-cals a day, and a total of about 1,200 calories a day. On them, a woman should be able to lose at least two pounds a week, a man at least three.

The sandwich diet feature

The feature of the sandwich diet is that it is popular, quick, economical, and self-regulating. I say popular because we are a sandwich-oriented society. Quick, because sandwiches lend themselves to variety and speed, with a number of ingredients able to be kept on tap in the refrigerator for days on end. Economical, because bread is still one of our lowest priced foods and the "innards" of a sandwich can be selected to fit any budget. Self-regulating, because the physical confines of the space between two pieces of bread are fairly rigid and less likely to be stretched than plate servings.

Of course, let it be understood right here and now that we are not talking about hero sandwiches or any other kind of colossal rolls or special bread sizes that are now coming into vogue.

When we say sandwich, we mean for you to use the average size loaf of bread and the standard rolls on which we will elaborate later.

How Phyllis lost 10 pounds fast

I remember one client for whom the Sandwich Diet was "made to order." Phyllis, at 32, was recently divorced. She was the mother of two young children and ten pounds above her most attractive weight.

For some time, she had managed to keep off at least some of the offending ten pounds by a daily intake of amphetamines. But the side effects of these "diet pills" began to take their toll. She suffered from palpitations, taut nerves, and other uncomfortable symptoms.

Those ten pounds were just enough to push her from an 8 to a 10, a size that she flatly refused to buy. She was very conscious of her extra poundage, almost neurotically so. She found herself shunning social functions and beach parties, especially among her inner circle of friends whom she described as "disgustingly slender and able to eat anything they want any time."

Phyllis was a sandwich eater and had always been so from a child. She would rather eat sandwiches than any gourmet dish and consequently was totally unable to follow any established diet. Needless to say, she was enthusiastic about my sandwich diet. It was a "natural" for her.

As is often the case, some modification in the existing eating habits can accomplish the desired effect without drastic changes. It certainly proved so with Phyllis, for within a few weeks those ten unwanted pounds were gone, and so was the mental load she carried because of them.

How to Make a Delicious Sandwich
That Is Piled High with Nutrients

If you cannot tolerate a high protein diet, then you must elevate the carbohydrate content of your daily fare at the expense of protein.

Just how far can you go in eliminating protein? Remember, this is the one food that your body is not able to synthesize out of other foods. And yet it is the most important maintenance food that your body requires.

This body requirement runs roughly between 300 and 400 prote-cals a day. Toward the lower figure if you are smaller in stature, and also toward the lower figure if you are getting on in years.

The sandwich diet consists of three sandwiches, or their equivalent, a day. To get the minimum protein requirement, two of these must contain high protein ingredients such as eggs, cheese, poultry or meat.

Remember, when you are barely meeting your body's protein requirement, as you are on the Sandwich Diet, you are not likely to be risking symptoms of protein intolerance.

Protein must be joined by other basic body requirements. This means that we must not only choose nourishing ingredients for our sandwiches but we must select the most nourishing types of bread.

Carbohydrates As Empty Calories

Carbohydrates can be "empty" calories. That is, they provide energy or turn to fat but do not yield, of themselves, anything of nutritive value to the body.

Famous "Life Extension Specialist" Paul C. Bragg, 92 years young at this writing and still leading an athletic life, is a dynamic speaker and in demand all over the world. One of his most effective stage demonstrations is to take a loaf of white bread, tear it apart, and roll the inside into a ball.

Then he bounces the ball on the stage, and as it rebounds into the air, he roars, "That's the junk that puts the mounds of fat on you!"

How to know breads for nutrient value

Some breads are not empty calories. They are made with whole grains that have not been denuded of nutrients. Also, there are breads made with special seeds, flours, or fruits. Although some of these are slightly higher in calories, they are exceptionally higher in nutritive value. So the calorie increment more than pays off in nutritive advantage.

In ascending order, here are the more nutritious breads:

Poor: White, bagels, white rolls, English muffins, frankfurter and hamburger rolls.
Better: Enriched white, rye, cracked wheat, seed rolls.
Good: Date nut loaf, pumpernickel, protein and health breads.
Best: Wheat germ, whole wheat.

What goes into these three sandwiches a day should also be selected for top nutritive value.

In ascending order here are the more nutritious sandwich fillers:

Poor: Packaged and processed meats, jellies, and jams.
Better: Cream cheese, peanut butter, canned fish.
Good: Hot or cold meats, poultry and fish salads.
Best: Greens, tomatoes, organ meats, eggs, cheeses.

The sandwich diet has a target limit of 1200 total calories per day.

The average bulging sandwich runs about 350 to 400 calories. To make it more bulging by adding lettuce and other greens cannot add any significant total to each sandwich—say 50 to 75 calories. Since some types of sandwiches run considerably less than 350 calories, even though you are a tower builder, you cannot do anywhere near the harm that can happen when a conventional diet is fractured by an extra portion.

The beauty of the sandwich diet is that we are psychologically attuned to a sandwich being a meal. And when it is a bulging sandwich, we are psychologically attuned to having enjoyed a big, satisfying meal.

Some Typical Days on Three Bulging Sandwiches

A sandwich for breakfast?

Hardly.

But you can see how a scrambled egg and two slices of bacon can fit on a piece of toast. Whether you place it on the toast and top it off with another piece of toast in sandwich fashion or eat them side by side is immaterial.

Breakfast can be such a sandwich or such a plate; eggs any style with bacon, sausage, or ham—toast on the side, or top and bottom. Or it can be a steak sandwich or chipped beef on toast.

Lunch can be a hamburger or frankfurter. Or you can make some tuna or salmon salad or egg salad. Peanut butter and the famous BLT (bacon, lettuce, and tomato) are popular choices.

If you cook a chicken, you can make hot chicken sandwiches with white meat and cut up the rest for several days of chicken salad sandwich lunches. Cheese sandwiches are just right for lunch—American, Camembert, Swiss—all of these popular cheeses are fine.

Always add a few leaves of lettuce, cabbage, or other greens to your luncheon and dinner sandwiches for added flavor and nutrients.

Come dinner time, you might want to make yours an open sandwich with hot meat. Whether you can add gravy or not depends on your calorie count for the day so far. (See sample menus below.) Gravy adds about 100 calories with little to no offsetting benefit in minerals and vitamins. But I must admit it dinner-fies a sandwich,—makes it more like the evening meal.

Sample Sandwich Diets for Weight Loss

Here are a few sample menus that might guide in extending your Sandwich Diet to at least 30 eating days of gratifying weight loss.

Day #1

Breakfast (270 calories):
  Two poached eggs on toast, black coffee or tea
Lunch (360 calories):
  Sardine (3 oz.) sandwich with lettuce, diet cola
Dinner (365 calories):
  Boiled tongue (4 oz.) sandwich with cole slaw, black coffee or tea
Total calories 995. Gravy may be added to the evening sandwich. Also
  a 5-ounce glass of milk or orange juice may be added to the menu.

Day #2

Breakfast (375 calories):
  Bacon (3 slices), cinnamon toast (2 slices), coffee or tea
Lunch (475 calories):
  Ham salad (3 oz.), ice tea
Dinner (300 calories):
  Chicken livers and mushrooms on toast, coffee or tea
Total calories 1,150. One-half grapefruit (small) permitted today.

Day #3

Breakfast (300 calories):
  Small steak on toast, coffee or tea
Lunch (330 calories):
  Grilled American cheese with lettuce and tomato, diet soda
Dinner (580 calories):
  Eggs Benedict (two eggs, Canadian bacon, Hollandaise sauce on
  English muffin), coffee or tea
Total calories 1,210. No extras permitted today.

Day #4

Breakfast (350 calories):
  French Toast (two slices), cinnamon and jelly, coffee or tea
Lunch (400 calories):
  Western sandwich, iced coffee
Dinner (410 calories):
  Roast lamb, pork, or beef sandwich (3 oz. meat or 2 oz. meat with
  gravy) with lettuce, coffee or tea

Total Calories 1,160. 5-oz. glass of unsweetened grapefruit juice can be added.

Day #5

Breakfast (325 calories):
Scrambled eggs (2), toast lightly buttered (2 slices), coffee or tea
Lunch (310 calories):
Roast lamb, pork or beef sandwich (2 oz.), diet cola
Dinner (400 calories):
Hamburger steak (3 oz.) on toast, spinach leaves, coffee
Total calories 1,035. Vegetable or salad with diet dressing can be added today.

Here are some additional do's and dont's in planning your menu:

- If you have calories to spare, do spend them on fresh milk, fruit, or vegetables.
- Toasting bread saves approximately 5 calories per slice. Do it freely if you wish.
- Adding a thin coat of butter or other spread adds 10 to 15 calories per slice. Don't, unless calorie count permits.
- Adding leaves of lettuce, cabbage, spinach, watercress, or similar greens adds negligible calories but considerable nutrients. Do use these in sandwiches regularly.
- Do favor proteins as your main sandwich ingredients—eggs, cheese, poultry, fish, or meat. Occasionally nuts are acceptable.
- If only one piece of bread is used, as in an open sandwich, credit yourself with 60 calories. Do use it for fresh dairy or produce.
- Do consider some mineral, vitamin supplement with your doctor's permission.

How to Add Variety to Your Bread
by Baking It Yourself

There was a time when you could tell that grandmother was baking bread two blocks away. Today, bread baking is a forgotten art, and even when an enterprising housewife does bake a loaf, it is a comparatively modernized, sanitized, and mechanized process.

If you have never baked a loaf of bread in your own kitchen, try it. It adds a home touch like a family reunion. Your first try is likely to be a taste treat compared to the average bakery or restaurant product.

One of the reasons housewives gave up making bread is that the process of kneading dough was a time consuming one, in addition to stove time. Kneading alone takes only ten minutes or so and that's not bad when automatic timers on ovens release you for other chores.

Here is the basic recipe for bread (materials are for one medium size loaf):

Three cups of whole wheat flour
Two tablespoons of butter
One teaspoon of salt
One tablespoon of sugar
One-half cake of yeast (or package)
One cup of milk

Warm the milk, add the yeast, sugar, and salt and stir well. Add the flour slowly, mixing thoroughly. About halfway through, melt the butter, add it to the dough, and continue adding the flour as you mix.

Stir and mix until dough is thoroughly blended. Then place on cutting board that has been lightly dusted with flour (hands, too) and knead dough back and forth until elastic to the touch. Place in a bowl in a warm spot and let rise to double size. Puncture to deflate several times. Now knead for several more minutes, shape into a loaf and place in a buttered bread pan. Let rise again to double size. Bake in a moderate oven, 350° to 375°, until brown—about 45 minutes.

Any basic cookbook will give you ways to make different style loaves and rolls as well as variations using cinnamon, onion seeds, etc.

Here are recipes for four breads that can add nutrition as well as interest and zest to your Sandwich Diet.

IMPORTANT: These contain approximately 30 calories per slice more than average breads. Either cut slices approximately one-third thinner or make appropriate adjustments in your calorie count.

Carrot Bread

2 cups whole wheat flour	2 tsp. vanilla
2 tsp. baking soda	13 oz. crushed pineapple
2 tsp. cinnamon	2 cups grated carrots
1/4 tsp. salt	1 cup chopped almonds
3 eggs	3/4 cups raisins
3/4 cup oil	3/4 cup dried apricots
3/4 cup buttermilk	1/2 cup chopped Brazil nuts
1/2 cup sugar	1/4 cup sunflower seeds

Mix all together and bake 50 minutes at 350°.

Indian Bread

1 cup whole wheat flour	1/2 cup water
1 tbs. butter	1/4 tsp. salt

Cut butter into combined salt and flour until thoroughly mixed. Add enough water to make pliable dough. Break off pieces the size of an egg and place on oiled tray. Cover with damp towel and leave for 1 hour. Roll into circles about 8 inches in diameter on floured surface. Cook on hot grill until dark golden brown, turn once. (For four.)

Cornmeal Bread

3/4 cup cornmeal	1 egg beaten
3/4 cup whole wheat flour	2 tbs. melted butter or oil
1 tsp. soda	1 cup sour cream
1 tsp. salt	1/2 cup milk
3 tbs. brown sugar	

Mix liquids and stir into mixed dry ingredients. Place in flat pan about 8 x 11 inches and bake at 400° for about 15 minutes.

Banana Bread

1/3 cup shortening	2 eggs
1/2 cup brown sugar	

Cream together, add eggs and beat.

1 3/4 cups sifted whole	1/2 tsp. salt
wheat flour	1 tb. gelatine powder
1 tsp. baking powder	1/2 tsp. baking soda

Sift together. Add to above mixture alternately with 1 cup mashed bananas combined with 1/2 teaspoon vanilla. Stir in 1/2 cup chopped walnuts. Pour into well-oiled loaf pan. Sprinkle with sesame seeds and bake for 45 minutes at 350°. Remove and cool on rack.

How to Substitute a Cocktail Party
for a Sandwich

We have given you five recipes for home baked bread. Actually, there are scores of varieties of breads in the cookbooks and in the supermarket.

The lowest calorie breads are the gluten-free diet variety. They have nearly half the calories. However, it depends what you add in the place of these saved calories as to whether you are doing yourself a favor. Add nothing, you lose faster. Add gravy, you deprive your body of more valuable nutrients.

Here's a winner for Sandwich Diet losers: You can substitute crackers for bread.

This opens up new vistas for the cocktail set. Crackers and dips may be substituted for dinner if your elbow is so inclined.

Use the calorie charts on the pages ahead to identify the type of bread or cracker at the party. Most popular brands are listed.

Each meal allows 120 calories for bread. This means you can substitute that many calories of party cracker, for dips or spreads.

For instance, your hostess has set out a cheese dip and Ritz crackers. You are counting the party as your dinner. You have clocked yourself at breakfast with 325 calories and at lunch with 375 calories. This leaves you with 500 calories for the cocktail party which you have chosen to call your dinner—and still stay under 1,200 calories.

Each Scotch on the rocks which you are drinking assuming one-ounce shots, is 85 calories. Set your drink limit at one, two, or three. Multiply by 85 and subtract from 500 for your canapé allowance:

500 Calorie Party Allowance

Number of Straight Whiskey One Ounce Shots	Calorie Allowance for Canapés
1	415

Number of Straight Whiskey One Ounce Shotes	Calorie Allowance for Canapes
2	330
3	245

A cheese sandwich is about 330 calories. So if you decide on two drinks, you can have in canapés the equivalent of a cheese sandwich. Since the sandwich assumes 20 calories of bread and since a Ritz cracker is 18 calories, you can dip into the cheese spread seven times.

Agreed this is a good deal of arithmetic but when you count calories, as you must do on high carbohydrate diets, you must be prepared to play this number game.

Choose From One Hundred Varieties of Breads, Rolls, and Crackers

The same process of computing calorie equivalents can be used to switch to rolls, buns, and muffins.

If a roll you select is less calories than two pieces of bread (120 calories), you can have more than one roll. But very likely not two. You will have to use part of a roll in proportion to the calories available. Another choice is to add fresh fruit or vegetables to compensate you for the difference.

At any rate, the sandwich diet can be varied by the use of these other bread products.

One young woman complained to me that she was sick of hamburgers for lunch and cheeseburgers for dinner, though she had lost 15 pounds in six weeks. She said she didn't like any other kinds of sandwiches.

I didn't try to talk her into any other kind of sandwiches. Instead, I told her to buy matzoh, English muffins, and sesame rolls. Then, to vary her hamburgers by using different fillers such as chives, finely chopped tomatoes, onions, peppers, garlic, or celery in different proportions. Oregano, soy sauce, pepper, rosemary, thyme, and basil are some of the different spices and herbs that can be added, I told her.

I suggested that the cheeseburgers could be varied by these same methods, also by changing the types of cheeses used—Cheddar (thinly sliced), jack, American, and Muenster are some that go well with hamburgers.

When another six weeks had passed, she had reached her weight goal but said she was enjoying her sandwich diet so, she was going to stay on it a while longer.

Suggestions to Vary Your Sandwich Diet

The following list of breads, crackers, rolls, and other bread-type products will give you some ideas of how to vary your Sandwich Diet and still stay within its 1,200-calorie limit. Trade names are used only as a recognizable guide, not an endorsement. Other products by various manufacturers may also be obtainable as similar to brands mentioned.

B R E A D—1 Slice   CALORIES

Corn and Molasses (Pepperidge Farm)	63
Cracked Wheat (Pepperidge Farm)	66
Gluten (Thomas' Glutogen)	35
Oatmeal (Pepperidge Farm)	66
(Profile)	52
Protein (Thomas' Protogen)	45
Pumpernickel (Pepperidge Farm)	79
Raisin (Thomas' English)	66
Raisin cinnamon, (Pepperidge Farm)	76
Raisin, cinnamon (Thomas')	63
Rye (Pepperidge Farm)	88
Wheat Germ (Pepperidge Farm Hovis Golden Sandwich)	58
White:	
(Daffodil Farm)	58
(Pepperidge Farm—large)	70
(Pepperidge Farm—Sandwich)	64
(Pepperidge Farm English Tea Loaf)	71
(Thomas')	64
(Wonder)	64
Whole Wheat (Pepperidge Farm)	61
Whole Wheat (Thomas')	65

B R E A D S T I C K S–1 Piece

Plain, (Stella D'Oro) 40
Onion flavored (Stella D'Oro) 36
Sesame (Stella D'Oro) 38

R O L L S–1 Piece

Biscuits, refrigerator, baked (Borden's Big 10 Flaky) 83
Biscuits, buttermilk, refrigerator, baked (Borden's) 57
Biscuits, sweetmilk, refrigerator, baked (Borden's
Southern Style) 57
Rolls:
Hard, brown and serve, baked, (Pepperidge Farm Club) 96
Hard, brown and serve, baked, (Pepperidge Farm Hearth) 54
Hard, brown and serve, baked (Wonder) 80
Hard, w/sesame seeds, brown and serve, baked (Pepperidge
Farm Sesame Crisp) 63
Soft, (Pepperidge Farm Dinner) 58
Soft, refrigerator, baked (Borden's Gem Flake) 70
Soft, onion-flavored, refrigerator, baked (Borden's
Onion Crescent Flaky) 95

C R A C K E R S–1 Piece

Bacon flavored (Nabisco Bacon Thins) 11
Barbecue flavored (Chit Chat) 14
Barbecue flavored (Sunshine Barbecue Snack Wafers) 17
Butter-flavored:
   (Hi-Ho) 17
   (Keebler Butter Thins) 17
   (Keebler Club) 15
   (Keebler Townhouse) 19
   (Nabisco Butter Thins) 15
   (Ritz) 18
   (Tam-Tams) 13
Butter-cheese flavored (Ritz Cheese) 18

C R A C K E R S–1 Piece *(cont.)*   **CALORIES**

Caraway (Caraway Crazy) 15
Cheese-flavored:
   (Cheese Nips) 5
   (Cheese Tid-Bits) 4
   (Cheez-It) 6
   (Che-zo) 5
   (Keebler Cheese Wafers) 11
Chicken-flavored (Chicken In A Biskit) 10
Ham-flavored (Hamies) 12
Matzo–1/2 Sheet
   (Goodman's Square) 55
   (Goodman's Tea) 37
   (Horowitz-Margareten Oven Crisp) 62
   (Manischewitz Regular) . . . . , . 60
   (Manischewitz Egg 'N Onion) 56
   (Manischewitz Tasteas) 68
   (Manischewitz Thin Teas) 54
   (Manischewitz Whole Wheat) 62
   (Manischewitz Egg) 68
Onion-flavored (Nabisco French Onion) 11
Onion-flavored (Onion Funion) 16
Oyster:
   (Dandy) 3
   (Keebler) 3
   (Oysterettes) 3
   (Sunshine) 4
Saltines, Soda and Water Crackers:
   (Crown Pilot) 73
   (Keebler Export Sodas) 25
   (Keebler Salt-Free) 14
   (Keebler Saltines) 14
   (Keebler Sea Toast) 61
   (Keebler Whole Wheat Sea Toast) 58
   (Krispy) 12
   (Premium) 12
   (Royal Lunch) 55
Sesame (Keebler Sesame Bread Wafers) 21
Sesame (Meal Mates) 22
Sesame (Sesame Sillys) 16

C R A C K E R S–1 Piece *(cont.)*   **CALORIES**

Sesame Cheese flavored (Sunshine Sesame Cheese Snacks) 16
  (Sociables) 10
Toasts and Toasted Crackers:
  (Dutch Rusk) 61
  (Holland Rusk) 38
  (Keebler Party Toasts) 15
  (Nabisco Zwieback) 31
  (Old London Melba Toast Rounds) 9
  (Old London Garlic Melba Toast Rounds) 9
  (Old London Pumpernickel Melba Toast) 16
  (Old London Rye Melba Toast) 16
  (Old London Salty Rye Melba Toast Rounds) 8
  (Old London Sesame Melba Toast Rounds) 11
  (Old London Wheat Melba Toast) 16
  (Old London White Melba Toast) 16
  (Old London White Melba Toast Rounds) 9
  (Sunshine Toasted Wafers) 10
  (Sunshine Zwieback) 30
  (Uneeda Biscuit) 22
Tomato-onion flavored (Sunshine Tomato-Onion) 15
Triangle Thins 8
Wheat (Keebler Wheat Toast) 15
Wheat (Nabisco Wheat Thins) 9
Wheat, shredded (Triscuit, Wafers) 22

Sandwich Diet Calorie Counter

The following list of sandwiches and their calorie content assumes a 120-calorie count for the two slices of bread used. Adjust the value if your sandwich breads or rolls are more or less. Toasting subtracts ten calories for each sandwich; butter or mayonnaise, lightly spread, adds about 25 calories per sandwich.

SANDWICHES

(MADE WITH TWO SLICES OF BREAD)

Item	Portion	Calories
American Cheese	2 med. slices used	330

Item	Portion	Calories
Bacon and Egg	2 med. slices & 1 egg	327
Bacon and Lettuce	2 slices ea. used	232
Bacon and Tomato and Lettuce	2 slices used	235
Barbecue Beef	2 oz. beef used	250
Barbecue Pork	2 oz. pork used	310
Bologna	2 slices used	360
Calf's Liver	3 oz. used	250
Camembert Cheese	1 triangle used	215
Cevelat	2 slices	230
Chateau Cheese	2 oz. pc.	330
Cheddar Cheese	2 oz. used	356
Cheese and Olive	1	350
Cheeseburger	1	500
Chicken Liver	3 oz. used	285
Chicken salad	3 oz. used	210
Chicken, Sliced	2 slices	205
with gravy		398
Club +	3 decker	575
Corned Beef	2 oz. beef used	250
Crabmeat	4 oz. meat used	280
Cream Cheese	2 oz. used	342
and Nut		400
and Jelly		442
and Olives		392
Denver, Western	1 med. egg used	400
Egg, Fried	1 med. egg used	230
Egg Salad	1 med. egg used	265
Frankfurter	1 med. used	254
Ham		
Baked	1 lg. slice	395
Boiled	3 oz. sliced	468
Fried	3 oz. slice	472
Luncheon Meat	3 oz. sliced	388
and Swiss Cheese	3 oz. ham	
	1 oz. cheese	538
Ham Salad	3 oz. used	474
Hamburger	1½ oz. gr. beef	288
Lettuce and Tomato	1 tomato and 4 leaves of lettuce	167
Liverwurst	2 slices	430
Meat Loaf	1 lg. slice	450

Item	Portion	Calories
Oyster, Fried	1 lg. used	242
Pastrami	2 med. slices used	300
Peanut Butter	2 tbs. used	330
with Jelly	2 tbs. used	500
Pimento Cheese	2 oz. used	334
Pork Chop	1 chop used	423
Pork Sausage	4 oz. used	470
Roast Beef	2 oz. beef used	310
with gravy		420
Roast Pork	3 oz. used	414
with gravy		510
Roquefort	2 oz. used	304
Cheese spread		334
Salami	2 slices used	360
Salmon		350
Salmon Salad	3 oz. used	370
Sardine	3 oz. used	358
Shrimp Salad	1 sandwich	200
Shrimp, Fried	6 medium used	230
Sole, Fillet of	4 oz. fish	208
Steak	1 sandwich	300
Summer Sausage	2 slices ¼" thick	230
Swiss Cheese	3 oz. sliced	445
Tongue	4 oz. sliced	365
Tuna	3 oz. used	280
Tuna Salad	4 oz. used	330
Turkey	4 oz. sliced	448
with gravy		600
Vienna Sausage	4 oz. used	374

Keys to Successful Weight Loss
on Three Sandwiches a Day

The sandwich diet will work for you if you work with it. It is a well-balanced regimen for those who cannot tolerate a high protein program. Here are its keys to success:

- Eat three sandwiches a day, no more, no less.
- Count your calories; stay within 1,200 a day.
- Pile on all the lettuce, cole slaw, or other greens you want.

- Use up left-over calorie allowances with skimmed milk, fruit or fruit juices, and vegetables.
- Vary bread, rolls, and crackers to avoid boredom.
- Limit beverages to coffee, tea, and diet sodas unless calorie margins permit.

10

THE RICE REDUCING DIET

The second diet I offer those of you who cannot tolerate a high protein fare is based on a food that is keeping one-third of the world's population slender.

In China, the word rice is the same word used for culture or agriculture. It is literally synonymous with farming. Rice is the staff of life not only for China but Japan, Indonesia, Malaysia, India, Thailand, Cambodia and large areas of the Soviet Union and the mid-east.

Few people realize that rice is grown extensively in the United States.

The big rice-producing states are Arkansas, Louisiana, Texas, Mississippi, and California.

In 1971, American farmers produced over eight billion pounds of rice. It is probably the finest rice in the world. Certainly, it is grown and harvested under the most mechanized and quality controlled conditions. Whereas other countries put some 400 man-days of labor per acre in growing and harvesting rice, American rice farmers need only two man-days per acre.

American rice is milled and refined but then there is a Federal requirement that certain minerals and vitamins be put back into the product to restore the nutritional value to its original whole grain level. This rice is called enriched, but a more accurate word would probably be restored

Rice Benefits

Enriched rice is fortified with iron, thiamine, and niacin.

Rice is largely carbohydrate. Eight ounces of boiled white rice contain 200 calories. Of these, 160 or 80 percent are carbo-cals. Some 12 percent are proteins and 8 percent fat.

Although limited, the protein content of rice is superior in amino acid structure to wheat and other grains because it contains all eight of the essential amino acids, and in proper proportion. For a protein to be utilized effectively, these eight amino acids must be present and in balance. It is possible that the over supply of one amino acid in a protein can reduce the utilization of another amino acid so that an efficient metabolizing of the protein occurs.

You don't have to be concerned about this when you eat a number of different proteins in ordinary foods. But it does become an important factor when, say, rice is depended on as the chief food in a diet—as it is in the rice reducing diet I am about to give you.

In research conducted at the University of Arkansas by Dr. Barnett Sure, it was reported that proteins in rice are superior to those in corn and oats and 158 percent better than wheat flour.

There is much to say for even the quality of the minimum fat content in rice. Most of it, 80 percent, is the preferred unsaturated fatty acid. The low fat content of rice and the fact that it is unsaturated fat makes rice highly accepted by physicians for use in low fat, low cholesterol diets.

There are other nutritional advantages to rice. There are appreciable amounts of phosphorus, also of iron.

And it digests easily and completely.

Rice Is Easy on the Delicate Digestive System

Doctors prescribe rice for a number of health situations. I find it an ideal diet food when health problems dictate certain precautions. See what your doctor says.

Rice requires very little work by the digestive system to utilize its energy and nutrients. In fact, rice takes only an hour to digest under normal conditions, compared to the two to four hours needed by other foods.

That is one of the reasons hospital dieticians make frequent use of rice in the regular diet, the light diet, the soft diet, and variations needed by special patients.

Other reasons are that rice is termed a non-allergenic food. That is, few people ever have hypersensitive reactions to rice. Rice flour is often used in place of wheat flour when an allergy can be traced to wheat.

Rice is a bland food, so it is useful in hospital cases of indigestion, ulcers, cardiospasm, and other problems involving the gastro-intestinal tract.

Rice is easily masticated by the aged. It is economical, easily prepared, as familiar as potatoes, and a versatile, esthetic food.

So much for the build up. Now where's the hitch?

The Hitch to the Rice Diet

The hitch is that the Rice Reducing Diet is not a permissive diet. There are no eat-all-you-want items on it. It has all the disadvantages of the standard diet I pointed out in the first chapters of this book.

But if you have to go on a carbohydrate-high diet, this is one of the best.

Another hitch: Rice must be cooked properly or it loses half of its nutritive ingredients. The problem is water. Some people like to rinse rice before cooking and again after cooking. Rinsing, as well as cooking in too much water, can divest the rice of 80 percent of its thiamine, half of its riboflavin, and more than half of its niacin.

Advantages of brown rice

Brown rice is more nutritious than white rice. It is the same rice only it has not been "de-enriched" as thoroughly as the white rice. That is, it is not quite as refined. What happens is that in the milling process the rice grains are cleaned to remove chaff, dust, foreign matter, etc. Then the husks are removed from the grains. Now you have brown rice. Only the outer hull and a small amount of bran have been removed. The rice in this stage has a slightly more chewy texture and a delightful nut-like flavor. It is preferred by many people.

When additional layers of the bran are removed, the white becomes whiter in color and you have the standard "polished" white rice.

When you buy rice, try the brown variety on your diet first. It is more nutritious per calorie. If you must buy the white, consider these two types:

- Parboiled rice is milled by a steam and pressure process that gelatinizes the starch in the grain and aids in the retention of natural vitamin and mineral content. After cooking, parboiled rice tends to be fluffy with the grains more separate and plump.
- Pre-cooked rice is milled as usual, then cooked. After cooking, the moisture is removed through a de-hydration process. Pre-cooked rice requires a minimum of preparation time as it merely needs to have the moisture restored and heated. One advantage is that pre-cooking is done with a minimum of water so that here again the fullest nutrition of the grain can reach your plate.

Seven Days on the Rice Reducing Diet

If you would like to check out the Rice Reducing Diet for one week, I recommend that you tailor the menus to total no more than 1,200 calories.

At this level, women should lose two pounds a week, men about three pounds a week.

I have used some menus and recipes supplied by the Rice Council of America[1] and find that my clients enjoy them as well as succeed with them in losing weight.

I list seven days of the Rice Council menus here together with a few recipes referred to in the menus. These menus have been prepared by the staff of the Rice Council under the supervision of Mrs. Dorothy F. Hutcheson, Institutional and Consumer Director, with menus developed by Mrs. Rae C. Hartfield, ADA, registered dietician.

---

[1]P.O. Box 22802, Houston, Texas 77027.

SUNDAY

(Total Calories 1194)

Breakfast:
Orange Juice (1/2 cup)	55
Sunnyside Rice	170
Bacon (1 slice)	47
Coffee Tea	
	——
	272

Mid-morning:
Milk (skimmed—1 cup)	90

Lunch:
Rice Garden Salad	102
Spinach (½ cup) with	20
Hard-cooked Egg (1)	80
Canned Apricots (3-4 halves)	66
(unsweetened or in light syrup)	
Coffee Tea	
	——
	268

Mid-afternoon:
Bouillon or Consommé (1 cup)	10

Dinner:
Broiled Steak (4 oz.)	240
Toasted Onion Rice (½ cup)	132
Green Asparagus Spears (6 stalks)	20
Sliced Tomatoes Vinaigrette	30
Blueberries	
(Fresh or frozen—½ cup)	42
Coffee Tea	
	——
	464

Bedtime:
Milk (skimmed—1 cup)	90

MONDAY

(Total Calories 1192)

Breakfast:
Prune Juice (½ cup)	85
Puffed Rice (½ cup) with	23
Sliced Banana (½)	44
Sugar (1½ tsps.) and	25
Milk (skimmed—½ cup)	45
Whole-wheat Toast (1 slice)	55
Coffee Tea	
	——
	277

Mid-morning:
Milk (skimmed—½ cup)	45

Lunch:
Spanish Rice Salad	99
Boiled Ham (2 ozs.)	170
Fruited Orange Gelatin (½ cup)	86
Coffee Tea	
	——
	355

Mid-afternoon:
Bouillon or Consommé (1 cup)	10

Dinner:
Lamb and Rice Skillet Dinner	297
Broiled Peach Half	33
Coleslaw (½ cup)	50
Citrus Fruit Cup (½ cup)	35
Coffee Tea	
	——
	415

Bedtime:
Milk (skimmed—1 cup)	90

TUESDAY

(Total Calories 1126)

Breakfast:
Melon Balls (frozen—½ cup)	55
Poached or soft-boiled egg (1)	80
Whole-wheat Toast (1 slice)	55
Butter or Margarine (½ tbs.)	50
Coffee Tea	
	——
	240

Mid-morning:
Milk (skimmed—1 cup)	90

Lunch:
Dried Beef with Rice	154
Italian Zucchini (½ cup)	30
Pear-Cottage Cheese Salad	92
(1 pear half and ¼ cup cottage cheese)	
Coffee Tea	
	——
	276

Mid-afternoon:
Bouillon or Consommé (1 cup)	10

Dinner:
Homestead Chicken and Rice	298
Broccoli (½ cup)	26
Chef's Salad with Low Calorie Dressing	30
Cranberry Frappé (½ cup)	66
Coffee Tea	
	——
	420

Bedtime:
Milk (skimmed—1 cup)	90

WEDNESDAY
(Total Calories 1183)

Breakfast:

Grapefruit Juice (½ cup)	50
Hot Cooked Rice (½ cup) with	90
Milk (skimmed—½ cup) and	45
Sugar (1½ tsp.)	25
Canadian Bacon (1 slice)	85
Coffee Tea	
	___
	295

Mid-morning:

Milk (skimmed—½ cup)	45

Lunch:

Rice and Crab Casserole	177
Dilled Green Beans (½ cup)	23
Rye Bread (1 slice)	55
Fresh Fruit Cup (½ cup)	70
Coffee Tea	
	___
	325

Mid-afternoon:

Bouillon or Consommé (1 cup)	10

Dinner:

Liver Fricassee over Rice	303
Cauliflower with Lemon (½ cup)	15
Pineapple-Paprika Twist on	
Lettuce (1 slice pineapple)	40
Lime Sherbet (¼ cup)	60
Coffee Tea	
	___
	418

Bedtime:

Milk (skimmed—1 cup)	90

THURSDAY
(Total Calories 1184)

Breakfast:

Orange Juice (½ cup)	55
Cottage-fried Egg (1)	
(using ½ tsp. butter or margarine)	95
Toast (1 slice)	55
Butter or Margarine (1 tsp.)	35
Coffee Tea	
	___
	240

Mid-morning:

Milk (skimmed—1 cup)	90

Lunch:

Chicken and Rice Ring with	
Tomato Aspic	215
Cooked Cabbage (½ cup)	20
Orange Sherbet (¼ cup)	60
Coffee Tea	
	___
	295

Mid-afternoon:

Bouillon or Consomme (1 cup)	10

Dinner:

Beef-Julienne with Asparagus	380
Seasoned Yellow Squash (½ cup)	17
Head Lettuce Wedge (1/6 head) with	
Low Calorie Dressing	22
Minted Pineapple (½ cup—water pack)	40
Coffee Tea	
	___
	459

Bedtime:

Milk (skimmed—1 cup)	90

FRIDAY
(Total Calories 1205)

Breakfast:

Grapefruit-Orange Segments (½ cup)	55
Mushroom Omelet	
(2 eggs—1 tsp. Butter or margarine)	185
Toast (1 slice)	55
Coffee Tea	
	___
	295

Mid-morning:

Milk (skimmed—1 cup)	90

Lunch:

Rice Tuna Salad Ole!	204
Corn on the Cob (1 ear)	
(with 1 tsp. butter or margarine)	100

Sliced Peaches (½ cup)	35
(fresh, frozen, or canned, unsweetened)	
Coffee Tea	
	___
	339

Mid-afternoon:

Bouillon or Consommé (1 cup)	10

Dinner:

Stuffed Fillet of Sole with Shrimp Sauce	245
Braised Carrots and Celery (½ cup)	25
Country Style Cucumber-Onion Rings	25
Fruited Lime Gelatin (½ cup)	86
Coffee Tea	
	___
	381

Bedtime:

Milk (skimmed-1 cup)	90

(Total Calories 1191)

Breakfast:	55	*Mid-afternoon:*	
Grapefruit (½)	90	Bouillon or Consommé (1 cup)	10
Hot Cooked Rice (½ cup) with	45	*Dinner:*	
Milk (skimmed—½ cup)	25	Chicken Vermouth with Rice	319
Sugar (1½ tsp.)	95	Tomato-Lettuce Salad with	
Bacon (2 slices)		Low Calorie Dressing	40
Coffee Tea	——	Strawberries (½ cup) with	
	310	Low Calorie Whipped Topping	45
		Coffee Tea	
			——
			404
Mid-morning:			
Milk (skimmed—½ cup)	45		
Lunch:		*Bedtime:*	
Luncheon Pancakes with Chinese Sauce	229	Milk (Skimmed—1 cup)	90
Seasoned Green Beans (½ cup)	23		
Carrot Sticks (½ carrot)	10		
Fresh Fruit Cup (½ cup)	70		
Coffee Tea			
	——		
	332		

Sunnyside Rice

(Calories per serving: 170)

¼ cup chopped onion
¼ cup chopped green pepper
1 tablespoon butter or margarine
6 eggs

2 cups cooked rice, salt and pepper
    to taste
2 tablespoons grated Parmesan cheese

Sauté onion and green pepper in butter until tender but not brown. Add rice and seasonings. Cook until hot.
Make 6 indentations with back of a spoon. Break an egg into each indentation. Sprinkle with cheese. Cover and cook until eggs are of desired doneness. Serve with slices of broiled tomatoes, if desired. Makes 6 servings.

Rice Garden Salad

(Calories per serving: 102)

2 cups water
2 tablespoons tarragon vinegar
2 chicken bouillon cubes
1 teaspoon salt
1 cup uncooked rice
½ cup diced cucumber (peeled
    and seeded)

¼ cup finely chopped green pepper
2 tablespoons thinly sliced scallions,
    including green tops
¼ cup diced pimento
¼ teaspoon freshly ground black pepper
½ cup yogurt

Combine water, vinegar, bouillon cubes, and salt in a saucepan. Bring to a boil. Add rice and stir well. Cover, reduce heat and simmer 15 minutes, or until rice is tender. While hot, add cucumber, green pepper, scallions, pimento, and black pepper. Toss lightly but thoroughly. Spoon into a 1-quart lightly oiled mold. Chill several hours. To serve, unmold on plate and garnish base with a ring of cucumber slices. If desired, surround mold with tomato slices, serve with yogurt. Makes 6 servings.

Toasted Onion Rice

(Calories per serving: 132)

1 cup uncooked rice
1 package (1-3/8 ozs.)
   dehydrated onion soup mix
2 cups boiling water

1 can (4 oz.) sliced mushrooms, drained
1 tablespoon butter

Place rice in shallow pan. Toast at 400 degrees, stirring occasionally, until golden. Add remaining ingredients. Cover; reduce temperature to 350 degrees and bake 25 to 30 minutes longer. Makes 6 servings.

Spanish Rice Salad

(Calories per serving: 99)

3 cups uncooked rice
  (cooked in fat free chicken
   broth)
1 cup diced green pepper
1 cup chopped celery

3 tablespoons minced onion
¼ cup chopped pimento
½ cup low calorie Italian dressing
4 tomatoes, peeled and quartered

Combine rice, green pepper, celery, onion, and pimento; mix well. Chill. When ready to serve, pour dressing over rice-vegetable mixture. Toss lightly. Spoon onto salad plate and surround with quartered tomatoes. Makes 8 servings.

Lamb and Rice Skillet Dinner

(Calories per serving: 297)

1-½ pounds boneless lamb
  shoulder

1-½ cups fresh or frozen peas
2 tablespoons minced parsley

1 clove garlic, split
1 tablespoon butter or margarine
2 tablespoons minced onion
½ cup diced celery
½ pound (2 medium) tomatoes

1-½ teaspoons salt
¼ teaspoon pepper
¼ teaspoon basil
1-¾ cups water
¾ cup uncooked rice

Remove fat from meat and cut into small cubes or slices. Brown meat and garlic in butter in large skillet. Remove garlic. Add onion and celery and cook 5 minutes or longer, stirring frequently to prevent over-browning.

Remove skin from tomatoes and cut into small pieces. Add to meat. Bring to a boil. Lower heat; cover and simmer about 30 minutes or until meat is tender.

Add remaining ingredients in order listed. Again bring mixture to a boil and lower hear. Cover and simmer about 20 minutes, or until rice and peas are tender. Makes 6 servings.

Dried Beef with Rice

(Calories per serving: 154)

½ cup chopped onions
1 cup chopped green pepper
2 tablespoons butter or margarine

1 jar (2½ ozs.) sliced dried beef,
   chopped
3 cups cooked rice

Saute onions and pepper in butter until soft but not brown. Add dried beef; cook 2 to 3 minutes. Add rice and continue cooking until thoroughly heated. Makes 6 servings.

Liver Fricasse over Rice

(Calories per serving: 303)

1-½ pounds beef liver, cut into
   long strips
2 tablespoons vegetable oil
   or shortening
1/3 cup sherry

1 teaspoon salt
¼ teaspoon pepper
1 clove garlic, crushed
3 cups hot cooked rice
1 can (1 lb. 4 oz.) stewed
   tomatoes

Brown liver on each side in oil. Add wine and simmer gently for 5 minutes. Add remaining ingredients except rice. Cover and continue to simmer for 45 minutes or until liver is tender. Remove cover and allow sauce to thicken if necessary. Serve over hot cooked rice. Makes 6 servings.

Rice and Crab Casserole

(Calories per serving: 177)

1 pound crab meat (fresh, frozen or canned)	¾ cup grated carrot
1 can (4 ozs.) sliced mushrooms with liquid	2 eggs, beaten
	½ cup skim milk
2 cups cooked rice	½ teaspoon seasoned pepper
1 package (1 3/8 ozs.) onion soup mix	¼ teaspoon thyme
	Paprika

Combine all ingredients. Spoon into a buttered 1½ quart casserole. Sprinkle with paprika. Bake, covered, at 350° for 30 minutes. Makes 6 servings.

Homestead Chicken and Rice

(Calories per serving: 298)

3 broiler-fryer breasts, halved	1 teaspoon paprika
1 teaspoon seasoned salt	1 heavyweight large brown grocery sack
½ teaspoon garlic salt	
¼ teaspoon seasoned pepper	Rice

Clean and dry chicken. Combine seasonings and sprinkle over chicken. Arrange chicken in sack, forming a single layer. Close sack opening, securing with paper clips. Place on foil-lined baking pan and bake at 375° for 1 hour. Serve with rice. Makes 6 servings.

Mushroom Rice

1 cup uncooked rice	1 can (2½ ozs.) sliced mushrooms with liquid
½ cup sliced green onions (with tops)	2 cups chicken broth (fat free)
1 tablespoon butter or margarine	½ teaspoon salt
	¼ teaspoon seasoned pepper

Place rice in baking dish. In skillet, saute onions in butter until soft. Add remaining ingredients. Bring to a boil. Pour over rice; stir. Cover with tight fitting lid or foil and bake at 375° for 25 to 30 minutes.

Chicken and Rice Ring with Tomato Aspic

(Calories per serving: 215)

2 cups diced cooked chicken	3 hard-cooked eggs, chopped
2 cups cooked rice	1 tablespoon lemon juice
2 cups sliced celery	1½ teaspoons salt
½ cup finely chopped green onions	1 teaspoon seasoned pepper
1 can (10½ ozs.) mushroom soup	2 cans (10½ ozs. each) tomato aspic, chilled

Combine chicken, rice, celery, and green onions; toss lightly. Add soup, eggs, lemon juice and seasonings. Blend well. Spoon salad into a 1½ quart ring mold which has been coated with a light film of mayonnaise or salad dressing. Pack down tightly, pressing with back of spoon. Bake at 350° for 25 minutes. Unmold and serve with diced tomato aspic in a chilled bowl in center of ring. Makes 8 servings.

Beef Julienne with Asparagus

(Calories per serving: 380)

1½ pounds boneless round steak	1/8 teaspoon pepper
2 tablespoons butter or margerine	1½ cups beef broth
1 clove garlic, minced	¼ cup cornstarch
3 tablespoons minced onions	1/3 cup water
1 12-ounce package frozen cut asparagus	1 can (4 ozs.) sliced mushrooms with liquid
2 teaspoons salt	3 cups hot cooked rice

Cut meat into strips about 3 inches long and 1/8 inch thick. Sauté meat, garlic, and onions in butter over high heat, stirring constantly, until meat loses its red color. Add asparagus, salt, pepper, and beef broth to skillet and bring to a boil. Lower heat; cover and simmer 8 to 10 minutes, or until asparagus is just tender. It should not be over-cooked. Blend cornstarch with water. Add to beef-asparagus mixture together with mushrooms. Cook until thickened and clear. Serve over hot rice. Makes 6 servings.

Stuffed Fillet of Sole with Shrimp Sauce

(Calories per serving: 245)

1 cup diced celery	1 teaspoon salt
1 cup sliced onions	¼ teaspoon pepper
1 tablespoon butter or margarine	1½ pounds sole fillets
3 cups cooked rice	Shrimp Sauce
2 tablespoons diced pimento	

Saute celery and onions in butter until tender. Add rice, pimento and seasonings. Turn into a buttered 2-quart shallow casserole. Arrange fillets on top of rice. Season with additional salt and pepper. Bake at 375° for 25 minutes. Serve topped with Shrimp Sauce. Makes 6 servings.

Shrimp Sauce

2 tablespoons cornstarch	¼ teaspoon basil
1½ cups chicken broth (fat free)	½ teaspoon garlic powder
1 can (4 ozs.) sliced mushrooms with liquid	12 shrimp, peeled and sliced in half lengthwise

Combine all ingredients and cook over low heat, stirring constantly until thickened.

Luncheon Pancakes with Chinese Sauce

(Calories per serving: 229)

3 cups shredded cabbage	2 teaspoons salt
½ cup finely chopped onions	¼ teaspoon pepper
2 cups cooked rice	2 tablespoons soy sauce
8 eggs, beaten	Chinese sauce

Combine cabbage, onions, and rice. Add salt, pepper, and soy sauce to beaten eggs. Stir into cabbage mixture. For each pancake pour 1/3 cup mixture on a lightly greased griddle. Cook until brown on each side. Serve with Chinese Sauce. Makes 15 pancakes (3 per serving).

Chinese Sauce

1½ cups chicken broth (fat free)   1 tablespoon soy sauce
1 tablespoon cornstarch   salt and pepper to taste

Mix together chicken broth and cornstarch. Cook until thickened. Stir in soy sauce and seasonings.

Chicken Vermouth with Rice

(Calories per serving: 319)

3 pounds choice broiler-fryer   1 medium onion, thinly sliced
   parts   12 cloves garlic, peeled
2½ teaspoons salt   2 tablespoons chopped parsley
½ teaspoon pepper   1/3 cup dry white vermouth
3 medium carrots, sliced   ¼ cup sour cream
2 ribs celery, thinly sliced   Baked Rice

Dry chicken. Sprinkle with salt and pepper. Place all ingredients except the sour cream and rice in a 2-quart casserole. Cover. Bake at 375° for 1½ hours. Remove from oven; stir in sour cream. Serve over Baked Rice. Makes 6 servings.

Baked Rice

(Ideal for any oven meal!)

1 cup uncooked rice
2 cups boiling chicken broth (fat free)
½ teaspoon salt

Combine ingredients in a buttered casserole. Stir once. Cover with foil or a tight fitting lid. Place in a 375° oven for 30 minutes before chicken is done.

Rice Tuna Salad Olé!

(Calories per serving: 204)

1 can (6½ ozs.) chunk tuna (water   1 teaspoon salt
   pack), drained   ½ teaspoon Tabasco

2 cups cooked rice
¼ cup finely chopped onion
1 tablespoon vegetable oil
2 tablespoons vinegar

2 tomatoes, finely diced
1 small head lettuce, finely
   shredded
2 cups corn chips (regular
   size)

Break tuna into bite-sized pieces. Stir in remaining ingredients except corn chips. Chill. At serving time add corn chips and toss lightly. Makes 6 servings.

Of course, any substitutions can be made to vary the above seven-day fare as long as the calorie equivalents are maintained. You can cross carbohydrate and protein lines as this is not a no- or low-carbohydrate diet. But try to stay with a minimum of 25 percent protein calories to satisfy the body's requirements.

There is no crossing calorie boundaries, though,—if you want the diet to work.

The Crash Program for Reducing with Rice

If you'd like to up your weight loss by a pound or two per week, you had better be ready to make some sacrifices.

Models who need to knock those last few stubborn pounds off have had excellent results with this crash program. So have the roly-polys.

One of the reasons why a strict diet succeeds with rice as its backbone is that rice acts as an expander for food. It magnifies the number of times you put a forkful in your mouth, chew and swallow. It absorbs the flavors of meats and complements them. You feel that you are eating more.

However, nothing in this chapter should be construed to mean that you can survive on a diet of rice alone. You need fruits, vegetables, meat, eggs (or else. . . .).

In 1972 the U.S. Public Health Services published the findings of a nutritional survey of Laos villagers, conducted by the Thomas A. Dooley Foundation and the University of Hawaii. Only about half the children born survived childhood. (In the United States 90 percent survive childhood.) Malnutrition was prevalent among 50 percent of the children. The researchers found goiters, bulging stomachs, skin lesions, and physical deficiencies in iron, calcium, vitamin A, and riboflavin. Surprisingly, their diet of rice appeared to provide adequate protein, thiamin, and niacin probably due to its being under-milled, home-pounded rice.

You must supplement rice with protein and other foods from the dairy, fruit, and vegetable categories. Remember, your body cannot manufacture protein from other types of food. Nor can it produce minerals and vitamins from thin air. These are needed not only to function on a healthy and vital level but they are needed to burn fat. The metabolizing of your own fat is a complicated process that utilizes an imposing array of nutrients.

Here is your total allotment of food for one day under this crash program. "Divvy" it up into three meals any way you like. I'll give you a typical day of menus in a minute. Note that there is enough rice—one and one half cups for three rice portions a day. So you can have rice for all three daily meals.

Here is the way it adds up:

Crash Program with Rice

1-½ cups (cooked) white rice
   The rice may be boiled in water or fruit or vegetable juices.
4-ounces of poultry, ground round steak, or veal
                          or
4-ounces of fish. Select from bass, bluefish, cod, flounder, haddock, halibut, mackerel, or trout.
1 pint of skimmed milk (2 8-ounce glasses)
1 fruit from Group A
2 fruits from Group B
1 cup vegetable from Group A. (*Note:* No canned vegetables should be used.)
1 cup vegetable from Group B
Do not use bouillon cubes, catsup, celery salt, celery flakes, chili sauce, salad dressings, garlic salt, horseradish with salt, mayonnaise, meat tenderizer, meat extract, mustard, olives, onion salt, pickles, relishes, soya sauce, Worcestershire sauce.
Use salt extremely sparingly.

Fruits, Group A

1 cup grapegruit sections, fresh or canned, unsweetened
6-ounce glass of grapefruit juice, unsweetened

1 medium size orange
6-ounce glass of orange juice
1 cup papaya cubes
1 cup fresh strawberries

Fruits, Group B

1 small apple
½ cup unsweetened applesauce
2 fresh apricots
4 halves dried apricots (uncooked)
½ small banana
½ cup fresh blackberries
½ cup fresh blueberries
¼ cantaloupe
10 dark sweet cherries
2 dates
2 fresh or dried figs
½ grapefruit
¼ cup grape juice
½ cup Malaga, Tokay or
    Thompson seedless grapes

1 wedge honeydew melon, 7" x 2
1 cup cubed watermelon
½ mango
1/3 medium size papaya
1 medium size peach
1 small pear
½ cup cubed fresh pineapple
1/3 cup unsweetened pineapple
    juice
2 medium size fresh plums
2 tablespoons seedless raisins
½ cup red raspberries
1 tangerine
1 cup tomato juice

Vegetables, Group A

Asparagus, 6 spears
Broccoli
Carrots
Collards
Escarole
Green Beans

Lettuce
Pumpkin
Tomatoes
Turnip greens
Winter squash

Vegetables, Group B

Bean sprouts
Brussels sprouts
Cabbage
Cauliflower
Celery
Chard
Cucumbers

Endive (Belgian)
Kohlrabi
Mushrooms
Okra
Radishes
Summer squash

Here is one day, just as an example of how the diet works:

Breakfast

Orange juice—6-ounce glass
Boiled rice with skimmed milk, cinnamon—½ cup
Coffee, skimmed milk or black

Lunch

Asparagus—6 spears
Boiled parsley rice—½ cup
Fresh berries—½ cup
Skimmed milk—8-ounce glass

Dinner

Broiled ground round steak—4 ounces
Boiled curried rice—½ cup
Brussels sprouts
Peach or tangerine
Coffee, skimmed milk or black

Night Cap

Skimmed milk—5-ounce paper cup

Reference is made to parsley and curried rice. Parsley rice is made by merely adding one teaspoon of dried minced onion to the liquid in which the rice is cooked and then adding two tablespoons of minced parsley to the hot cooked rice.

Curried rice is made by adding one teaspoon of dried minced onion and two teaspoons of curry powder to the liquid in which the rice is cooked.

Rice Can Squeeze Excess Water from Your Body

Special diets produce special effects. Certain individuals, usually women, have a water retention problem. The body becomes bloated with water. Since sodium helps the body to soak up water, they not only have to be concerned with protein, carbohydrates, and fats but must turn their attention also to their intake of sodium.

How Christina overcame her retained water weight

Christina was a case in point. She could literally put on two pounds from one bite of a delicious half-sour pickle. Persons with Christina's problem must avoid foods such as pickles, relish, catsup, pickled, cured or smoked meats, or fish, celery, olives, salt, monosodium glutamate and many other foods, herbs and spices containing high intensities of sodium.

I requested her physician's permission to put her on my Rice Alone Diet. He agreed and the next day Christina began the monotonous, but dramatically effective, diet of rice. As a result, in two days she lost nine pounds! In one week she had dropped 13 pounds!

This diet, originally conceived at Duke University, is effective primarily because it contains no sodium. Consequently, by a process of dehydration excess water in the body tissues is lost rapidly. However, before attempting this diet, as with other diets in this book, consult your physician to make sure that it will have no ill effects on your particular body chemistry.

Telltale signs of excess water in the tissues are puffiness in the body joints such as fingers, knees, and ankles. The medical term is edema. Many physicians test for this condition by pressing their finger against the skin and watching the skin return to its normal contour. If the time is prolonged for the skin to return fully, edema is suspected.

Rice Alone Diet—This diet produces a dramatic weight loss through dehydration. Rice contains no fat and only a trace of sodium. It is intended to reduce fluids in the body tissues. The diet is simple, can be tolerated for a number of days, but should be undertaken only with the permission of and under the supervision of your physician.

Boil ordinary white or Minute Rice in unsalted water. Wash rice before and after boiling—eat as desired. Allowable beverages: any non-caloric liquids.

This is just one more plus in favor of the rice diet. If I had to vote for the most effective high carbohydrate diet, there is no doubt that I would give the nod to. . .

Rice.

11

THE PRECISION POINT SYSTEM
FOR SLOWING OR ACCELERATING
YOUR WEIGHT LOSS

Most people can eat all they want and will lose weight on the Free Diet (Chapter 3).

Even more people will enjoy all the food they want and lose weight on the High Protein Diet (Chapter 4).

Those who don't will certainly lose weight without hunger on the Higher Protein Diet and Highest Protein (Crash) Diets (Chapter 5).

This same progression, applied to people, can also be applied to the amount of weight they will lose.

However, it will be different for everybody.

A man may begin to lose weight on the Free Diet, then stop. He may shift to High Protein Diet and lose only a half pound a week. When he tries the Higher Protein Diet, it may still not hit a pound a week. Does this mean he must go on the Crash Diet? No, there is a way of enjoying the permissiveness and wide choices of the High and Higher Protein Diets and still be able to accelerate your weight loss to a gratifying number of pounds per week.

The secret is in quantity control combined with protein control.

How the Precision Point System Works

On the Precision Point System, you still have the High, Higher, and Highest Protein Diets.

However:

1. You must be selective in choosing high protein foods.
2. You must limit quantity intake.

You are asked to choose your protein foods based on their protein percentage. These protein percentages are listed in the tables of protein, fat, and carbohydrate values in Chapter 6. The center column (column four from left or right) lists the protein percentage of every food with the highest percentage at the top of each category.

Suppose you are planning your week's menus prior to shopping. You are on the Higher Protein Diet and you want to use the Precision Point System to accelerate your weight loss. You see by the table below that meats on the Higher Protein Diet must exceed 49 percent protein. So you check the Chapter 6 tables under "Meat, Poultry, Fish, Shellfish, Related Products."

The list starts with a lean roast of beef and shows it to be 77 percent protein. That's great. Next come beef hearts at 68 percent and a few other beef cuts of 62 percent including broiled steak, lean only. Roast leg of lamb is also 62 percent.

All these are permissible as they are over 49 percent, the bottom percent limit for the Higher Protein Diet. However, you can go down the list only as far as veal cutlet, 49 percent. Corned beef at 47 percent is not permitted on the Higher Protein Diet nor is broiled steak with fat at 46 percent.

Similarly, some chicken is permitted, but some is not. You can go about half way through the fish list. The only cheese eliminated by the 20 percent limit is cream cheese.

Since most of these foods are free of carbohydrates, what you are doing is cutting down on fats so that a higher proportion of your intake is fat destroying protein.

Portions, Points, and Pounds

The second of the two steps of the Precision Point System for controlling your weight loss is to count your points.

I have applied a point value system to each category of food based on the energy in that food. This is the control factor. It enables you to eat more of the foods you like and cut down where the pleasure sacrifice is the least.

How is this different from counting calories? Well, although the points are broadly related to the calories, I'd rather you not get back into the habit of counting calories.

Carbo-calls should be counted. Calories, per se, no.

So that is why I prefer that those who want to pit weight loss against time get the hang of this Point System.

Here is how it works.

- Each food category has a point value per ounce or per other appropriate measure. For example, all meat is 10 points per ounce.
- You set your own total daily point allowance depending on how fast you wish to lose. For example, you may be losing 1½ pounds a week on 140 points daily. If you cut down to 120 points daily, you will lose about one-half pound a week more, or a total of 2 pounds a week.
- To lose more weight, you can shift to a higher protein diet, or you can cut points. To lose less weight, you can stay on the same program protein-wise and add points, or you can move to a lesser protein diet and maintain your point count as is.

Twenty points less = ½ pound a week faster weight loss.

Forty points less = 1 pound a week faster weight loss.

It's like setting an oven control to get the job done at the time you want it done, or as your physician wants it done.

On p. 210 is the Precision Point System Dieting schedule for your guidance.

A Crash Diet with Six Meals a Day

I have found that splitting a meal into two meals can reduce hunger tendencies and contribute to satisfaction. This becomes increasingly important on as rigid a program, albeit a temporary one, as the Point Crash Diet. Here is how it might work on a typical day:

Recommended daily points: 100 to 160. Minimum allowable: 80 (for temporary use only).

Food	Value Points	Required Protein % High Protein Diet	Required Protein % Higher Protein Diet	Required Protein % Highest Protein (Crash) Diet
Meat	10 per oz.	77-20%	77-49%	77-49%
Fish	6 per oz.	84-22%	84-50%	84-50%
Poultry	6 per oz.	70-42%	70-42%	70-42%
Eggs	7 each	33%	33%	33%
Cheese	10 per oz.	30-20%	30-20%	None allowed
Cottage Cheese	4 per oz.	78-52%	78-52%	78-52%
Skimmed Milk	7 per 8 oz.	40%	40%	40%
Salads	5 per generous portion	60-20%	40-40%	None allowed
	3 per small portion	1 generous portion daily	1 small portion daily	
Vegetables	5 per generous portion	60-20%	60-40%	None allowed
	3 per small portion	1 generous portion daily	1 small portion daily	
Fruits or Fruit Juices	6 per portion	20-10%	20-10%	None allowed
		1 portion daily	1 portion daily (no juice)	
Fats	10 per tablespoon	13-0%	13-0%	13-0%

Six Meals a Day on the Precision Point Crash Diet		Point Value
Meal 1	8 oz. skimmed milk or 2 oz. cottage cheese	7-8
Meal 2	1 egg or 1 slice of roast beef	7-10
Meal 3	1 scoop cottage cheese	12
Meal 4	1 individual can of tuna fish	18
Meal 5	4 oz. sliced chicken	24
Meal 6	3 oz. lobster salad with one tablespoon of mayonnaise	28

Note: Meals should be separated by approximately two hours. This is simply an example of a crash protein diet. You may duplicate other foods to approximately the same value. However, salad, vegetables, and fruits may not be used.

Louise Had to Knock Off 25 Pounds before the Big Day

Louise, a very attractive housewife of 41, 5'7" tall, and mother of two boys, had been referred to me by a former patient.

When she came for her first visit, weighing 198 pounds, she appeared quite disturbed. Her weight problem was of fairly long standing. She had undergone several years of psychiatric treatment for anxiety and depression caused by marital problems. She blamed these problems for her overeating and her desire for sweets and pastries.

Her son's bar mitzvah was to take place in less than three months, and she wanted very much to look as attractive as possible.

This was a short period of time to solve such a weighty problem but, determined to help her all I could, I put her on my Highest Protein Diet with instructions to use the Point System for precision weight loss,—in this case the limit being 100 points. In view of the fact that she was an active woman, she responded faster than most of my patients would have done. She lost weight consistently each week—just a few ounces up or down from a 2½ pound loss. By the time the big event arrived, she had lost 26 pounds and improved her appearance considerably.

This success had whetted her appetite for further weight loss. I relieved the stringency of her diet somewhat by putting her on the Higher Protein Diet. This raised her point limit to 120 points. She continued to lose about two pounds a week. In a few months, she approached her desired weight of 135 pounds. At that time, I changed her diet to the Protein Maintenance Diet (see next chapter) and she no longer needed to count points.

You Can Lose Weight by Eating More

The beauty of the point system is that you can continue to lose weight even by eating more. Unless you have an urgency, as Louise did, why lose three pounds a week when you can lose two pounds a week?

You are going to be slender a long, long time. Arriving at your weight goal a week earlier or a month earlier is less important than avoiding feelings of deprivation and "diet."

Slow weight loss is more likely to be permanent weight loss.

The closer you are to get to 80 points—the most rapid diet possible—the closer you are to starvation. Hence, it is not recommended for use for more than a few days at a time.

I'll wager you that the temptation will be great for highly motivated losers to cut to 80 points and not want to move back up. The reason is that you will not feel as hungry on a high protein fare as your carrot stick and melba toast colleagues.

When they are on a low calorie fare—but high in carbo-cals—they are triggering their pancreas to release insulin into the bloodstream, which lowers the blood's sugar and yields an irritable,

212 THE PRECISION POINT SYSTEM FOR WEIGHT LOSS

hungry feeling. Also, those carbohydrate foods are long out of their stomach when your protein foods are still giving you a satisfied feeling.

Still, 80 points are not enough to provide the kind of eating fun I want you to have.

Remember my basic precept: extreme diets invite the yo-yo syndrome. You end the extreme diet and you begin to gain back the poundage. Down and up. Down and up.

Who needs it? Rather take it slowly and surely.

Important Case Histories in Point

George got so taken with the comfort he experienced on 140 points that, even though he was losing two pounds a week on the Higher Protein Diet, he cut to 120 points, then 100 points. Now he was losing three pounds a week. He felt that the sooner he got to his goal weight, the sooner he could rejoin his colleagues at those long, two martini lunches. He was right. He saved himself three weeks. But the quick shift to the maintenance diet and unlimited points set him back ten pounds—or five weeks.

But then there was Hillary, described in the next case.

Stay within protein percentages or lose points not pounds

Hillary describes her relationship with food quite frankly.

"While I'm cooking dinner, I am always snacking, sampling, and munching. When the kids are home from school, it's more of the same."

During those rare times in her marriage when she had not been involved with kitchen chores, Hillary had no difficulty in maintaining the figure that she liked. But those times became even more rare as the number of her children rose to seven.

"If I could only stay out of my own kitchen," she laughed, "I wouldn't have any trouble."

Hillary was 22 pounds overweight. With her height of 5'1", and her small-boned frame, 22 pounds made her feel dumpy and middle-aged. She yearned again to feel slender and attractive.

She had joined a weight-watching group but instead of losing, she gained. This diet was approximately 1,200 to 1,400 calories and was reasonably high in carbohydrates.

I, too, had trouble getting Hillary's weight to respond. She started with the High Protein Diet at 120 points. After one week, she had lost nothing. The following week she used the Higher Protein Diet, also with 120 points. That week she lost only one-half pound.

Hillary was beginning to get impatient with herself and with me. So I cut her points further, and further. She did not begin to lose weight regularly until she reached 80 points. Then, she really began to lose.

Eventually, the story had a happy, slender ending. But there's a moral: Based upon her activities, including taking care of seven children, Hillary should have lost weight on 120 points. But for her this was still too much. She was eating out of habit and to join her children's fun. This meant that carbo-cals were creeping in and protein percentage was creeping down. If you are on a diet eating the right foods and you are not losing weight, you are eating too much—more than your stomach or your appetite dictate. If you are not eating too much, then you are eating the wrong foods.

Keep the protein percentage in mind as much as the points. Relax one, and it costs you the other,—or it costs you pounds.

How to Get the Most Nourishment Per Mouthful

We talked earlier about empty calories.

High protein foods are not empty calories. They are nourishing calories. Carbohydrate calories can be empty calories if they are devoid of minerals and vitamins.

Vitamins and minerals are as important to the well-being of the body as proteins are to the destruction of fat.

If you are on a limited point, high protein fare, you may be limiting vitamins and minerals. That is why I recommend that you take vitamin and mineral supplements according to your physician's instructions while on crash diet or Precision Point program.

However, you can also increase your vitamin and mineral intake by knowing what foods in each category are the highest in these nutrients.

This increase in nutrients costs you nothing in points. For instance, calf's liver is equivalent to "beef, lean" on the protein percentage table, being some 77 percent protein. Yet, a lean steak at 10 points per ounce does not give you anywhere near the minerals and vitamins of calf's liver at the same 10 points per ounce.

Furthermore, because calf's liver *is* so rich, a four-ounce portion will satisfy you as much as an eight-ounce portion of steak. You save 40 points for another meal.

All things being equal, the preference should be calf's liver.

But all things may not be equal. . .

For one thing, you may despise calf's liver.

For another, calf's liver may be rich in nutrients that your body needs less than some other particular nutrient, found in great abundance in say, eggs.

So I am now going to give you a brief run-down on what the various vitamins and minerals are, in what foods they are found, and the advantages to the body.

One advantage for all of them I state unequivocably, right here and now: minerals and vitamins help your body function properly. One of the activities in a properly functioning body is the destruction of excess fat.

Minerals and vitamins contribute, therefore, to the effectiveness of high protein foods as fat destroyers.

The Alphabetized Substance That Revitalizes Your Body

Back in 1912, a scientist named Funk was analyzing rice polishings in an effort to discover the ingredient in them which seemed to prevent beri-beri. The several substances he found he called vitamins. Since then, many more of these substances have been identified and, because of their complexity, they have been given letters rather than names. In one case, even the specific lettered vitamin B has been found to contain a whole family of different substances which have not been numbered.

A point to remember in your dieting

Be vitamin-aware. No matter what diet you are on, be judicious in your selection of vitamin-rich high protein foods. Fruits, vegetables, and salads are "go slow" foods in a high protein slenderizing program, but this is all the more reason to select your daily greens for their vitamin content as well as their diet balancing and taste value.

Meet your body-strengthening vitamin friends in the VITAMIN TABLE on p. 215.

VITAMIN TABLE

Vitamin	Deficiency Symptoms	Areas Benefited	Found In
Vitamin A	Deteriorating vision Night blindness Other eye problems Kidney stones Bladder stones Susceptibility to colds Susceptibility to skin infections Defective teeth or tooth enamel Digestive problems	Better digestion Increased resistance to infection Good vision Minimum of respiratory problems Delay in senility Vigorous cell growth Healthy skin	Butter Cheese Egg yolks Fish liver oil Turnip greens Dandelion greens Kale Spinach Broccoli Mustard greens Calf's liver
Vitamin B_1 (Thiamine)	Irritability Lack of concentration Beri-beri Retarded growth Fatigue Lack lustre hair Poor muscle tone	Appetite, muscle tone, heart rhythm—all improved Nerve tonic Hair beautifier	Soy beans Brewer's yeast Navy beans Lima beans Green peas Turnip greens Beef heart Beef kidney
Vitamin B_2 (Lactoflavin) (Riboflavin)	Fingernail problems Corneal vascularization Digestive disturbances Pellagra Nausea Insomnia Dizziness	Virility Fertility Good digestion	Beef liver Beef kidney Lean meat Turnip greens Brewer's yeast Green peas
Vitamin B (Niacin)	Diseases of the central nervous system Certain eye and skin conditions Pellagra	Normal metabolism, including oxidation of carbohydrates Growth in children	Red Salmon Lean meat Beef heart Beef liver Beet greens Spinach Cauliflower Soybeans
Vitamin C (Ascorbic Acid)	Susceptibility to infection Scurvy Wounds slow in healing Gum problems Listlessness	High resistance to infection Marrow produced for bones Prompt healing of mucous membranes	Citrus fruits Strawberries Cabbage Dandelion greens Turnip greens Mustard greens Broccoli Rose hips
Vitamin D	Irritability Weakness Bone and teeth deficiency	Enables body to absorb calcium from foods Helps normalize blood	Eggs Tuna Salmon Sunshine
Vitamin E (Tocopherol)	Muscular wasting Sexual activity	Muscle regeneration Sexual regeneration	Corn oil Soy oil Meats Brussels sprouts Spinach
Vitamin F (Fatty acids)	Tendency to arteriosclerosis	Proper blood cholesterol levels	Corn oil Soy oil Wheat germ oil
Vitamin K	Hemorrhaging	Proper blood coagulation	Tomato Cauliflower Cabbage Spinach

215

The above sources are only a partial list of the most common fat destroyer foods and other low carbohydrate sources. Consult nutrition books for additional sources.

How to Have a Radiant Body While You Lose Weight

I can always tell when people have been through the starvation diet wringer. Sure, they look thinner. But they also look washed out!

They are nutritionally depleted. Their body cells have paid a price. Skin, hair, and muscle tone are poor.

They would have been better off on a fast. At least, they would be resting their bodies instead of working them and depleting them to metabolize food of questionable restorative value.

Your body needs minerals to build and maintain bone, teeth, nails, hair, and muscle—the structure of the body. It needs minerals to maintain proper blood circulation and coagulation. It needs minerals for normal metabolism and the maintenance of healthy tissues.

Some five million Americans are said to be suffering physical and mental impairment due to iron deficiency. Dr. Louis F. Diamond, a University of California Medical Center pediatrician, has found that the majority of such victims are children and adolescents who too often "live" on snacks.

Fortunately, iron and other minerals are found in the fat destroying foods of this program. Following is a rundown of key minerals, what they do for you, and where to find them:

Mineral	Importance	Found In
Iron	Essential for blood, enabling it to carry oxygen to the brain and all parts of the body. Prevents anemia, helps to remove carbon dioxide from the body cells.	Beef liver ⌐ Egg yolk ⌐ Chicken Most meats Oysters ⌐ Avocados Celery Soybeans Spinach Turnip greens ⌐

Mineral	Importance	Found In
Calcium	Essential for bones and teeth, coagulation of blood, proper functioning nerves, muscles and vital organs. Plays a part in activating enzymes.	Egg yolk Seafood Most cheeses Olives Kale Cabbage Mustard greens
Sodium	Prevents excessive loss of water from tissues, aids digestion of fat destroying proteins, assists in the absorption of other minerals and in maintaining a proper balance between them.	Bacon Cheese Saltwater fish Salt
Phosphorus	Works like calcium and with it in maintenance of body structure. Important in metabolism of fats and carbohydrates. Guardian of healthy blood and muscles.	Lean meat Ham Dried beans Lentils Cheese Saltwater fish Poultry
Potassium	Heart functioning, muscle action, bowel evacuation. With nitrogen, important to glands and nerves.	Spinach Turnip greens Beet greens Lima beans Avocados
Magnesium	Activation of enzymes, elimination of toxins, nerve stability.	Most meats Apples Cabbage Most greens
Copper	Works closely with iron, especially important to liver and spleen.	Beef liver Lobster Oysters Shrimp Egg yolk
Sulphur	Important to hair, nails and bile. Used in protein metabolism.	All meats All fish Eggs Beans

These are not all the minerals the body needs. There are many more. But some are needed only in minute amounts and are not usually the cause of deficiency diseases.

Notice how often beef liver, leafy greens, and most meats appear as sources. They are permitted on every high protein diet as well as the Point System diets. It would be wise to make organ meats and leafy greens (turnip greens, beet tops, spinach, mustard greens, etc.) a regular part of your weekly shopping list.

One time when being lightweight is not too healthy is: when you are born. A long-term British study has shown that babies weighing less at birth than they should are more likely to suffer from educational and behavioral defects by the time they reach school age. More often than not, these lightweight babies are born to a mother with a protein or mineral deficiency.

Mineral deficiency is suspect in many diseases. From acne and anemia to tooth decay and tuberculosis, specific mineral deficiencies have been identified.

The problem is so complicated that specific mineral intake for specific purposes is usually abandoned in favor of the shotgun approach: eat many mineral-high foods and take general (multiple) mineral supplements.

Warning: Both vitamins and minerals can be kidnapped before the food you expect to contain them reaches your lips. . . .

How to Be Sure of Adequate Vitamin and Mineral Intake

Where do plants and animals obtain the minerals that our body needs? The answer is from the soil. But therein also lies a problem.

Modern American farmers use a chemical farming system. They plant the same few crops in the same soil year after year. To obtain fast growth they supplement the tired soil with synthetic nitrogen and other chemicals that, if they do provide minerals, do so in unnatural imbalance.

In European countries, where farming has been going on for many centuries, the farmers use natural methods of replenishing the soil. European vegetables taste better and are more nourishing to the people who live on them.

There are only two things you can do about it as an individual seeking mineral-rich vegetables:

1. Keep an eye out for organic or naturally grown produce.
2. Use cooking methods that preserve what minerals are in the produce you buy.

More and more supermarkets are adding natural food departments. These are likely to start with shelves of carbo-cals: whole wheat no-preservative breads, wheat germ, honeys, etc. However, they are getting into organically grown lettuce, ranch-raised chickens, and other mineral and vitamin "conscious" foods.

Ask at your local supermarket. If the answer is "no," at least you will have registered your interest and hastened the day when the supermarket will stock these more healthful foods.

If you live in, or near, rural areas, inquire among local farmers whether they know any farmer that uses organic methods. Organic meat, poultry, and produce may cost slightly more but are worth the difference, especially for high protein dieters who need to make every high carbohydrate food item score high in vitamins and minerals.

Cooking methods that we use daily can destroy vitamins, dissolve minerals, and de-nature even the most natural of foods. Compound these cooking methods with low levels of nutrients to start with and it is a wonder that more of us don't suffer from acute deficiencies.

How to Knock Out Minerals and Vitamins in Your Diet

There are three cooking and preparation factors that sound the death knell for minerals and vitamins.

1. High temperatures cause impairment.
2. Cooking water dissolves nutrients.
3. "Air" oxidizes and prevents body usage.

If you were a calcium mineral in a head of cabbage, you might meet your demise in all three ways. After being cut up for cooking, you may be exposed to the air too long. If that doesn't get you, you may be cooked too long at a high temperature. Or, you may be submerged in the cooking water and later be thrown down the drain.

This is why a mineral or vitamin will not have lived in vain, if the vegetable it is residing in is eaten raw while fresh.

However, there are cooking and handling methods that do less nutritive damage than others. Following is a vulnerability summary of the vitamins and minerals discussed above:

Vitamin and Mineral Summary Vulnerability Factors

	Water Soluble	Destroyed or Impaired by Heat	Oxidized by Exposure to Air
Vitamin A	X (also fat soluble)	X	X
Vitamin B_1 (thiamine)	X	X	
Vitamin B_2 (riboflavin)	X	X	
Vitamin B (niacin)	X		
Vitamin C (ascorbic acid)	X	X	X
Vitamin D	(only fat soluble)		
Vitamin E	(only fat soluble)		
Vitamin F (fatty acids)		X	
Vitamin K		X	
Iron	X		X
Calcium	X	X	X
Sodium	X	X	
Phosphorus	X	X	X
Potassium	X		
Magnesium	X	X	
Copper		X	X
Sulphur		X	X

How to Preserve Nutrients in Storing and Cooking

About half of the vitamins and minerals by name (not

necessarily by quantity) are adversely affected by exposure to air. Of course, if you were that calcium mineral in a head of cabbage, and you were in an outside leaf, you would suffer more from the air than an inside leaf. The longer you waited to be used, the more depleted you would get.

Even the calcium in an inner cabbage leaf gets "air sick" when turned into cole slaw and left to stand. Warm air playing over exposed surfaces oxidizes and depletes the life-giving nutrients of cabbage. The refrigerator helps somewhat. Covering helps some-what. But eating the cabbage when freshly cut is the only satisfactory answer.

Vitamin A and C are especially vulnerable to air. The vitamin C in citric fruits and juices deteriorates rapidly once the skin is removed from oranges or grapefruit or when the juice is left standing.

Here are some tips to preserve the vitamins and minerals in the food you buy.

Air

- Use as soon as possible.
- Refrigerate.
- Freeze quickly if reasonably prompt use is not expected. (Meat and fish only.)
- Keep covered or wrapped.
- Don't cut, slice, shred, etc. until ready to use or prepare.
- Once prepared, serve promptly.

Water

- Wash or rinse minimally.
- Use as little water as possible in cooking.
- Favor steaming or pressure cooking for least water.
- Save cooking water for soups or drink as is.

Heat

- Avoid frying.

- Favor baking over broiling.
- Bake at lower temperatures.
- Learn to enjoy rare meats and only slightly cooked vegetables.

Well, we've apparently drifted away from the Precision Point System for controlling your weight loss. But have we really? For this system to be fun for you and your body, you have to enjoy the limited quantities even more. You need to get more oral satisfaction out of eating less.

Also, your body needs to get more nourishment per mouthful when portions are reduced.

I want you to be happy on less food, if indeed you must get on a restricted Precision or Crash diet.

I want you to be as well nourished, if not better nourished.

I want you to look radiant, feel energetic, be more youthful as you lose pound after pound. You should know how to take those necessary steps now by applying the simple principles in this book.

12

HOW TO EAT OUT,
ATTEND PARTIES, END DIETING
AND STAY SLIM ALWAYS

A 32-year old mechanic loses 45 pounds in four months, with a corresponding drop of six inches at his waist, and is able to slide under a car once again.

A 28-year old housewife loses 24 pounds in three months and is able to get modeling jobs while her youngster is at school.

A 54-year old bookkeeper, whose ill health has threatened her job, loses 35 pounds in five months and gets a raise.

Now what. . . .

A year later is the mechanic sending a helper under the car for him? Is the housewife resigning herself to being only a housewife? Is the bookkeeper's figure interfering with her figures?

Yes, if they were on a standard "reducing" diet.

No, if they were on a high protein "diet."

I have put quotation marks around the word diet in the second place because it is really not a diet in the sense that the standard diet is a diet.

Except for the few days that you have been on the Highest Protein (Crash) Diet or for the brief period you may have chosen to go on the Precision Point System, you have been eating all you want.

When you eat all you want, there is certainly no diet in the standard sense to get off. At worst, you begin to eat more carbo-cal foods at the expense of prote-cal foods.

Hopefully, there's less satisfaction in such a switch than there is in staying slim permanently.

One is oral satisfaction.

The other is the satisfaction of being attractive to the opposite sex, healthier, more productive, more popular, and headed for a longer life.

Is that worth giving up just for the oral satisfaction of having a dish of ice cream instead of cold slices of roast beef?

It would be a disservice if I told you that, once you have rid yourself of that excess weight, you could return to a life of hot dogs, pizzas, candy, pie, cakes, and other munchy missiles of the carbohydrate bombardment.

You may be able to have a couple of pieces of toast with your morning eggs.

You may be able to have a baked potato at dinner.

You may even be able to have both.

It all depends. . . . how you let this book work for you.

The Key to Maintaining Your Proper Weight for Good

Some people reach their goal on the Free Diet (Chapter 3). Just by eliminating sweets and starches, they lose weight, and attain their proper silhouettes.

This means they are very prone to putting on weight from sweets and starches. To maintain their proper weight, they must remain scrupulous in their avoidance of sweets and starches.

The Maintenance Diet(s)

• So, the Maintenance Diet for those who lost their weight on the Free Diet is: the Free Diet.

Some people don't get to lose any significant number of pounds until they go on the High and Higher Protein Diets. They don't react that sensitively to a few carbo-cals, more or less.

• So, the Maintenance Diet for the ones who have proceeded as far as the High Protein Diet is also: The Free Diet.

• And the Maintenance Diet for those who have proceeded as far as the Higher Protein Diet is: the High Protein Diet.

All persons who were required to go to a Crash Diet or to a Precision Point Diet to reach their weight goal may also regress one step. . . .

• The Maintenance Diet for Highest Protein (Crash) Dieters, or anyone who reached his goal by the Precision Point Diets, is the Higher Protein Diet.

So your Maintenance Diet is one of these three: Free Diet, High Protein Diet, Higher Protein Diet, depending on how far you needed to cut carbo-cals and points to reach your satisfactory rate of loss.

This is just a rule of thumb. You may have been losing weight at a rate that made you impatient, so you shifted to a stiffer program, although that rate may have made the next guy quite happy. Or some time requirement may have affected your choice of diet.

The proof is in the pudding that you don't eat.

Try the Free Diet as a Maintenance Diet. At the slightest signal from your scale, switch to the High Protein Diet as your Maintenance Diet.

If the High Protein Diet permits you to regain, then the Higher Protein Diet is your Maintenance Diet.

You can experiment similarly with certain foods that you want to restore, like that morning toast or the dinner potato. Restore one at a time. If, after a week of that food the scale says yes, let it remain. Then try adding another.

I'll wager very few people can pass the third add-a-carbohydrate food test. Heed the warning of the handwriting on the scale gauge.

Psychological Pressures on You and How to Handle Them outside the Kitchen

You are slender. You are attractive. Then comes that problem with your spouse.

Psychological problems can take various turns. They can bring on skin rashes, ulcers, or unwanted habits. They can also produce a few unwanted turns in your profile if food is an inherent weakness.

Sandra's handling of her "big" problem

A happily married school teacher, Sandra had joined two weight-watching organizations. She had taken diet pills and tried every diet she read or heard about. It was always the same story: she gained back quickly whatever she was able to lose. She had sought psychological help, but was assured that she had nothing to be concerned about.

Sandra had weighed 116 pounds in her late teens; at 20, when she married, she weighed 135 pounds; when she came to me, after 15 years of marriage the scale showed 197 pounds!

Analyzing her own situation, she felt that the tensions of her profession and the necessity of having to control her anger in the classroom were responsible for her eating too much between meals. This was only part of the story. She was convinced that part of the cause of her overweight was also the faulty dietary habits carried over from her parental home (her mother weighed 400 pounds).

Sandra shifts gears and reaches her weight goal

No argument here. The need for a complete change in her eating habits was obvious. First, she went on the Highest Protein (Crash) Diet. It was a very drastic change, even if only for seven days. But her husband, also somewhat overweight, lent not only his support but joined her on this diet. At the end of a week, I put her on the Higher Protein Diet which gradually brought her weight down to 150 pounds.

Since her goal was 135 pounds, I then shifted her to the High Protein Diet. Within another four months, she had reached this goal.

At the present writing, Sandra has been on the Protein Maintenance Diet for more than a year. When I last heard from her, she assured me that she experienced no difficulty whatsoever in maintaining her weight. I was especially pleased to hear that one of the side effects of her more healthful way of eating was the fact that she seemed much less affected by the aggravations of a teacher's life.

Frequently, part of our procedure in treating overweight clients is an initial interview by a psychologist. This interview often discloses the inner reasons for eating and how food is being relied on for more than its share of satisfaction.

Some Case Histories of Psychological Pressures

Study several of these cases. See if you can spot the cause and cure of their over-interest in food:

Case 343 • A high school teacher's husband is neither warm nor responsive. Sexual relationships with him have turned dull and devoid of passion. Her 185 pounds keep her from seeking outside sexual relationships which she feels would jeopardize her marriage and bring rejection of her children.

Case 512 • A 42-year old man gained custody of his children because of his wife's infidelity. Ever since the divorce, he has been gaining steadily. He has a satisfactory relationship with one woman but still sees others. He has been able to give up smoking successfully, but his 240 pounds are more than he can cope with.

Case 527 • A housewife, 37, began to gain weight shortly after her first pregnancy when her mother-in-law moved into her home. The home then became the scene of heated conflicts between her husband and his mother as well as smoldering tensions within herself. She now weighs 185 at height 5'3".

Case 563 • A housewife, 41, is happily married but they have been having financial problems. Her husband nags her about her weight, but for health reasons. At 19, she weighed 115. In her thirties, she weighed in the 150 to 175 range. She now weighs 230.

Case 601 • An office worker, she weighs 177 pounds at 5'3". She claims her husband drives her to food. They have gone their separate ways within the marriage. She wants a divorce but he won't talk about it. He refuses to let her see a physician about weight loss, fearing she would then find another man

and leave him. She had a hysterectomy several years ago and
has also had circulation problems.

The Answers to the Foregoing Cases

Some of the above are easy to analyze for weight gain causes,
but one or two may be tricky. *Here are the actual findings:*

Case 343 — Fear of jeopardizing marriage is a likely smoke screen. She
needs excessive food satisfaction to compensate for missing
sexual satisfaction.

Case 512 — He is insecure about his masculinity ever since the supreme
put-down by his wife. Smoking was a personality crutch
that he no longer needed. But food is a security substitu-
tion he needs until his sexual confidence is restored.

Case 527 — Yes, it was the mother-in-law, but largely because the
patient was very passive and had great difficulty in being
assertive. This was the basic problem that had to be handled
as she was rationalizing it under the table while she
increased her food rations above.

Case 563 — Financial security is something that has "bugged" her since
she left the protection of her parents' home. This current
critical period has increased its pressure on her to enjoy the
security of a constantly full stomach.

Case 601 — Like the menopause, a hysterectomy is often a traumatic
experience for a woman because of the inference that it
takes away some of her femininity. It was apparently at the
root of both husband and weight problem.

Figure your own possible psychological hang-ups

These are examples of the kinds of life happenings that change
eating habits. The number of possible problems that could enter a
person's life and affect his menus is infinite. They defy prediction.
But they do not defy recognition.
And with that recognition comes the beginning of a solution.
It is always more effective to treat causes than symptoms. If
you have a nagging psychological need for food as some sort of

emotional compensation, you won't be likely to lose weight on a permissive diet because you will probably eat more than your body requires. And you won't lose weight on a restrictive diet because you'll be able to stay on it only so long and then "so long" to any pounds lost.

The key clue to identifying the psychological cause is to review what events or changes have taken place in the time period when the weight gain began.

Who or what came into your life?

What is your attitude toward that?

How is eating related to that attitude?

Entertaining, Eating Out and Staying Slim

Can you go to parties and not fracture your Maintenance Diet?

Suppose your Maintenance Diet is the Higher Protein Diet; can you enjoy a night on the town?

All drinking aside, the food aspect of these two questions evokes a decisive "yes!"

I'm going to leave the drinking part to you,—except for this parting "shot":

Warning on alcoholic beverages

Free of carbo-cals are rye, bourbon and Scotch whiskeys, rum, vodka, gin, and brandy. With water, ice, or sugar-free soda, they remain free of carbo-cals. Also low in carbo-cals are dry wines. So a martini is all right. Beer and most cocktails and highballs are taboo as their carbo-cals can climb well over an entire day's allowance.

The food question is easy to solve

Now back to food.

Eating out on the high protein diets is sheer joy compared to the pained expressions you see on the faces of conventional dieters when they look over a tempting menu. They wind up forgoing the Chicken Kiev and the Veal Cordon Bleu and ordering a salad.

You do just the opposite.

You enjoy all the fish and meat appetizers and all the entrees. You ignore the potatoes but you have a vegetable or salad. Most good restaurants make cheese platters available for dessert and include delicious imported varieties. Or, there is fruit.

Eating out pitfalls are the bread that sits in front of you while you wait, the breading they fry in and stuff with, the inevitable potatoes, and the sweet desserts.

If you are not having an appetizer to keep you interested until the entree arrives, ask for your salad first and unless others in your party wish to indulge, ask the waiter not to bring bread or rolls.

At other people's parties, you have to stick to the hot hors d'oeuvres or other cold meats and fishes. Cheese cubes are a popular cocktail party item. So are the pigs in a blanket, which are tiny frankfurters wrapped in bacon. Take a toothpick and stab a meatball.

I always find a protein snack or two at a party.

As to my own parties. . . .

Party Snacks You Can Enjoy with Your Guests

I mix water chestnuts, soy sauce, crisp bacon, ham cubes and mushrooms.

I fry pork in sesame oil and skewer it to a morsel of fresh pineapple.

I broil prawns with dry mustard and cheddar cheese. I make fondue bourguignonne by cooking tender morsels of beef in butter and oil, dipped in curry sauce (curry sauce—combine two table-spoons of curry powder, one pureed clove garlic, one tablespoon lemon juice, and two 10½-ounce cans of beef gravy; add additional seasoning if desired, heat and dip—delicious).

My guests enjoy my spicy cocktail wieners. (I mix mustard with spicy barbeque sauce, heat, dip and eat.)

One-inch pork cubes that have been mixed with salt, pepper, and garlic and baked in a 350 degree oven for one hour are dipped in taco sauce and bring me rave reviews.

For delicious mushrooms, I stuff them with cheddar cheese or clams, and chopped meat seasoned with Worchestershire sauce, Tabasco, fine herbs, or whatever.

I mix meatballs with ground ginger and soy sauce and bake them in a slow oven.

At my parties, there are turkey meatballs, veal meatballs, and lots of kebabs which can be arranged Hawaiian style.

There are eggs, stuffed with asparagus. There are tomatoes, stuffed with shrimp. There is tuna, mixed with anchovies and there are pâtés made with smoked salmon and liverwurst and shrimp and crabmeat and chicken livers and mushrooms, and there is gefilte fish.

There is avocado and crabmeat, sprinkled with lemon juice and crisp bacon. There is caviar mousse, clams in aspic. There is antipasto and melon with prosciutto.

Excuse me, I am getting ill.

How to Travel Without Acquiring Excess Baggage

Entertaining is easy compared to international traveling.

Somehow, where new taste sensations are available, moderation goes out the window and you go overboard.

Airlines might make a sizable profit if they charged all the pounds you gain for the return trip as excess baggage.

I see by the papers that diet luncheons are being served by various domestic and international airlines.

That's great, but of course the problem hits you after you hit the ground. It's a big problem in Italy, land of the pastas, less of a problem in Scandinavian countries where fish is the order of the day.

Fish can be a life-saver almost anywhere in Europe. If you feel cornered by flour-thickened sauces and broadening breading, ask at your hotel desk where you might find a good seafood restaurant. You may be guided to the Contented Sole or Wheeler's in London, La Marée in Paris or Corinto in Madrid. Ask for your order to be broiled instead of fried.

Broiling is available almost everywhere and just about any restaurant will prepare an entrecôte, similar to our minute steak.

Paillard is the name for veal, flattened and served with lemon. Veal is excellent in Europe and, of course, a great fat destroyer food when carbo-cals are kept away from it.

Cafeterias, smorgasbords and buffets put the reins squarely in your own hands as you can see what you put on your plate. With a jaundiced eye for fattening carbo-cals and an appreciative flat stomach for fish, meat, poultry, cheese, and eggs, you can skirt the items that are suspect.

I often carry a few cans of tuna fish, mushrooms, and asparagus to tide me over wnen the choice is either the kind of starchy meal I shouldn't eat or no meal at all. I also carry tea bags, instant coffee (in one portion envelopes), and individually packed sugar substitutes.

The key is to penetrate the language barrier and be as selective as you are at a fine restaurant in your home town. The tendency is to ask the waiter about a few items on the foreign menu that you cannot read. He probably knows a few words of English but they usually do not include the words starch, flour, sugar, breading, etc. Rather than make him uncomfortable, you take a chance and order. Out comes a pasta prepared just for you. So you eat it and *you're* uncomfortable.

Insist on talking to the manager or somebody else who speaks English, or ask to see the ingredients before they are prepared in the kitchen.

Less sugars, starches, bread crumbs, and other carbo-cal sources are used in Asian food than in Europe. If you can skip the rice, you've got it licked.

Exercising Common Sense Is Better than Exercising to Take off Weight

"Oh, well, let's have a hamburger, we'll burn it off bowling tonight."

Whether you are at home or traveling, the battle is against carbohydrates.

It is a continuing battle, and, of course, most of the battle is fought on home grounds.

The carbohydrate bombardment is insidiously convincing at times.

"Great, for quick energy."

"Essential carbohydrates that your body needs to function properly."

The energy-nutrient sales pitch for carbohydrate foods is no more worthy than a carnival con man's come-on.

How to Watch the "Foods for Energy" Weight Builder

Carbohydrate foods are junk foods, energy and nutrition-wise. You know by now that sugar is absorbed quickly into the blood stream, raising the normal blood sugar level (maintained by proteins) so that you get a temporary feeling of euphoria or "lift," the same as alcohol, coffee or other stimulants provide. But then comes the rush of insulin to normalize the blood sugar level. It can lower it even below normal and you get a "down" feeling.

Those who rely on sugary snacks for quick energy and who feel the effects of the "quick energy" wear off, hit the candy box or cookie jar again and again to repeat the sugar-insulin cycle.

The steady energy of protein is far superior to the energy crisis caused again and again by carbohydrates.

The fact that carbohydrates are usually junk foods nutrition-wise, too, was pointed up recently when a housewife led a one-woman crusade against the kind of foods being sold to children in vending machines. A Bloomington, Indiana, mother of four succeeded in getting school authorities to replace the traditional empty calorie candy bars, packaged cookies and cakes, cokes and potato chips with fruit, raisins, nuts, and orange juice, certainly a step in the right direction.

Active people are particularly susceptible to the "quick energy" argument. Golfers, bowlers, tennis players often feel that a dose of sugar will help their game, give them more energy. The reverse is usually true. A protein meal several hours before a match will insure a steady and more dependable supply of blood sugar than the see-saw effect that is touched off by that surge of sweet stuff.

Exercise is no excuse to indulge in a coke or other carbohydrate pick-me-up. You work off a few ounces and then add a pound.

Exercise common sense, instead.

Don't let anything swerve you from a protein path. With plenty of delicious eating, it's a wide, wide path. Better the path than you.

Famous Last Words: "One Piece of Pie Won't Hurt"

Just this once.

It sounds innocent enough.

But it sounds the death knell for a slender person's attractive silhouette.

Just this once is never just this once. It sets a pattern for repeated sorties into the forbidden world of carbo-cals.

Even if it really is just once, there can be a long lasting effect.

Once the body is forced to store excess calories—with no fat destroyer foods to burn them off—it manufactures fat cells.

Now, a fat cell isn't here today and gone tomorrow. A fat cell is a storage unit that is kept around awhile. If you dump fat, the fat cell does not disappear, it merely shrinks.

It is still there waiting to inflate you again at the least carbohydrate transgression.

That's why it is easier to regain fat that you once had than for you to create new fat from a virgin threshold of normal weight.

Hence: "I wish I could be like Darlene. She eats anything and everything and never shows it."

When you give up carbohydrates you may be giving up some familiar, sweet taste. But all you are really giving up is a little oral pleasure and a lot of fat, ugly pounds.

A friend of mind had a birthday party. Imagine my surprise and admiration when, hardly had the dinner begun, out came—not a birthday cake—but a birthday steak, festooned with candles.

You don't need the baker. You can have just as much fun with the butcher and the candlestick maker.

How to Recondition Yourself from Time to Time Against Carbohydrates

The carbohydrate bombardment bursts around you every hour of the day. You may have changed. But it doesn't know this.

Television commercials continue to blast away at you to buy what you no longer eat. The car radio, billboards, and solicitous friends take pot shots at you with promises of pleasure from treacherous carbo-cals. Your favorite lunch spot continues to display fresh pies on the counter in front of you, and an ice cream wagon ding-dongs at you as it goes by.

You have got to be deaf and blind not to feel the wearing away of your resolve under this steady bombardment.

To survive as a slender, healthy, long-lived high protein person, you have to reinforce your defenses from time to time.

I gave you a relaxation-visualization technique in an earlier chapter. It is worth repeating now as it can be your secret weapon against the Trojan Horse treachery of "Mom, look, I baked some hot cross buns" or "Helen, I brought you over some of the fudge I made this morning."

Remember? Step one—sit in a comfortable chair and relax.

Step two—visualize sweets and starches turning to fat as they move down your throat.

Step three—see yourself enjoying meat, fish, poultry, cheese, and eggs and looking vibrant, healthy, dynamic, and slender.

That's all there is to it. You have insulated yourself against more of the carbohydrate bombardment,—just how well and for how long depends on these factors:

- Thorough relaxation of body
- Peaceful tranquility of mind
- Expectation of insulative results
- Sharpness and real-ness of the visual image
- Time spent in imaging
- Frequency of practicing this insulation procedure

Any book on meditation, yoga, or self-hypnotism[1] will give you techniques for deepening your relaxation and quieting the mind.

Understanding how mental pictures program the automatic (subconscious) portion of your mind will help you to believe that the exercise will be fruitful and enhance your expectation.

Imaging common pictures like a watermelon, an apple, a chair gives you the knack of imaging in Step two and Step three.

Holding the image a few seconds is better than having just a fleeting picture, and repeating the exercise daily helps to keep you safely away from the brink of surrender to any tempting villains.

---

[1] *How to Reduce and Control Your Weight Through Self-Hypnotism,* Sidney Petrie with Robert B. Stone, West Nyack, N.Y.: Parker Publishing Company, Inc.

Outwit Carbo-cals by Using Your Old "Computer"

The automatic or subconscious mind is similar to an electronic computer. It behaves you as it is programmed to do. This programming is done through experience and repetition. If you eat pizza once and it tastes good, you will eat it again. Eat it often enough and you become programmed as a pizza lover.

Maybe that is how you are programmed now. But what's good for the pizza is good for the goose. Eat poultry, meat, fish, cheese, eggs as your main meals and in-betweens, too, and you program yourself with slenderizing high protein habits instead of fattening carbohydrate ones.

The above lines tend to program you to do just that. But it took you only five seconds to be exposed to their programming. When you put the book down, you may walk into the kitchen or the supermarket and be programmed for twenty times as long by the sights, sounds, and smells associated with sweets and starches.

So the few lines above are cancelled out by new programming.

The trick is to tune out unwanted programming. You do this by *knowing*.

Know what you want to accept in the way of sensory input. If the mailman hands you a letter that doesn't belong to you, you do not accept it.

Speed readers are able to go through a book in an hour. One factor that permits them to make such good time is that they know what they are looking for, what they expect to get out of it.

If you set priorities for your attention, you light up when those priorities appear.

Get excited by proteins. Get turned off by carbohydrates. Then you "see" the proteins but you pay less attention to the carbohydrates.

Advertisers, manufacturers, and packagers spend millions trying to gain entry to your mind.

Open your doors of perception to them if the message is protein.

Slam the door if it's sweets and starches.

Be Health Conscious Not Diet Conscious

Another programming to which you have been subjected is that you have to diet to be slim, and that to diet successfully you have to starve and deprive your body.

If you approach fat destroying foods as you would approach a diet, you are not going to get off that yo-yo string.

Know that diets are a thing of the past for you, that a new way of eating to lose weight is not temporary. The new fare is not an "affair" but a marriage.

You have found a new, slender life style.

It is a life of easier bending, stooping, lifting, and moving.

It is a life of walking with a spring in your step.

It is a life of smaller clothing sizes and greater styling.

It is a life of eyes of the opposite sex that look at you in passing.

It is a life where drab mornings and evenings become beautiful sunrises and sunsets.

It is a life of health, and sexual attraction, and popularity.

It is the life you were born to live.

Put these pictures in your consciousness.

See yourself not on a diet, but on a "live it."

"What's for Dinner Tonight?"

"What's this, dear, it's very good."

"It's chicken in cream sauce with chives."

"Fattening, isn't it?"

"Nary a carbo-cal."

Dinners are going to be better than ever and easier to prepare as you get to know the protein pages of your cookbooks.

The whole family, no matter what their tastes, will enjoy the succulent fishes, savory roasts, and satisfying poultry dishes that are served at dinnertime.

The whole family, no matter in what direction they travel during the day, will find taste pleasure in the scores of quickie lunches that contain "nary a carbo-cal."

The whole family, no matter how much importance they give to breakfast, will enjoy the stand-up cold deviled eggs or the sit-down steaming platters of bacon and eggs.

Know what interests you:

- Hot and cold meats; hot and cold fishes; domestic and imported cheeses; turkey, chicken and other poultry; and eggs every style—in short, fat destroying foods.
- One daily leafy vegetable rich in minerals and vitamins; one crisp, raw salad, one piece of fresh raw fruit or the fresh or frozen juice thereof.
- Foods that are fresh wherever possible and free of chemicals, prepared so as to retain their natural nutrients.

We will not say goodbye to hearty, enjoyable eating, but goodbye only to the sickly sweet and starchy carbo-cals.

It is a fare on which you can live longer and better.

Fare well. And—it will look well on you.

INDEX